COORDINATION BREAKDOWN MANAGEMENT IN SURGICAL UNITS

---

from understanding of breakdowns to their detection and prevention through system design

Svetlena Taneva, Ph.D.

Printed by CreateSpace, Charleston, SC.

ISBN-13: 978-1461111917
ISBN-10: 1461111919

Diss. ETH No. 19345
Diss. TIK No. 120

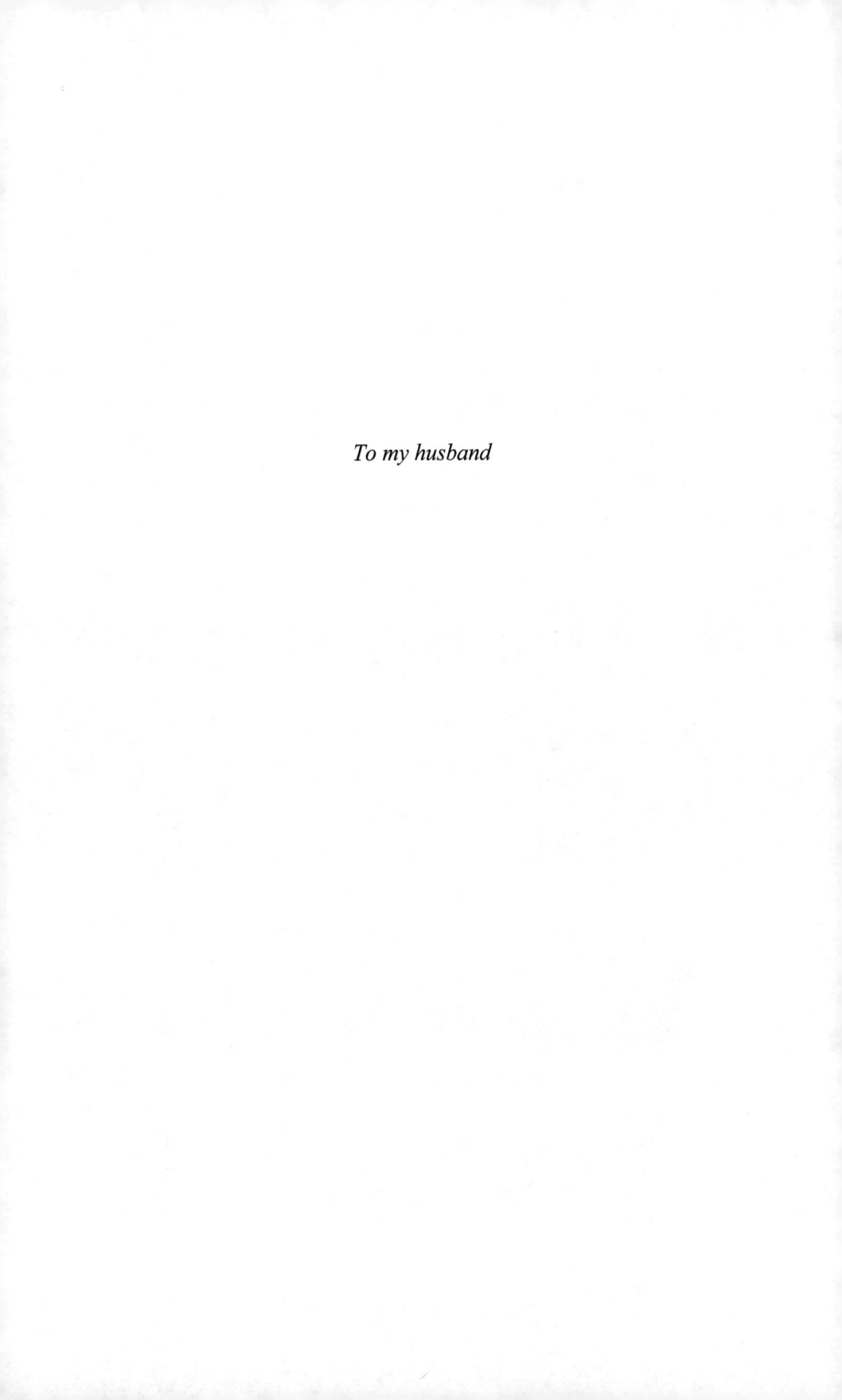

To my husband

Human error in medicine, and the adverse events that may follow, are problems of psychology and engineering, not of medicine.

John Senders, 1993

Acknowledgments

This work would not have been possible without the continuous support and guidance of Professor Dr. Bernhard Plattner. His input was the driver of this work.

My deep appreciation also goes to Dr. Anthony Easty and the Healthcare Human Factors team at the Centre for Global eHealth Innovation in Toronto – for supporting the research, facilitating the empirical work, and providing excellent guidance and a great learning environment.

For creating this great research opportunity and for her very insightful inputs through the years, I would like to offer special thanks to Dr. Effie Law.

I also extend my gratitude to Professor Dr. Gudela Grote for her advice, guidance, and constructive criticism that contributed to defining the quality of this work.

For their efforts in realizing the empirical work, I would also like to thank Jacqueline Higgins, Charlie Byer and the perioperative teams at both hospitals where the research was conducted.

Abstract

Communication and coordination breakdowns represent the leading cause of adverse events in healthcare, especially in the operating room environment – the wrong patient may be operated on, the wrong procedure may be performed, or consideration of specific patient information may be missed in surgery planning, preparation and execution. Across geographical and organizational boundaries, one in ten hospital patients becomes victim of a preventable adverse event – sometimes leading to death. As a response to such alarming reality of patients' prospects in a hospital, the patient safety discipline emerged in the 1990's.

One of the major research concerns in patient safety is the examination of the problem of communication and coordination breakdowns in the continuum of surgical patient care and the potential strategies for system and process improvement. Research has shown that breakdowns stem from an interplay of human errors, socio-technical system design factors, and poorly designed technology interfaces. However, the majority of research focuses on the narrow domain related to cognitive aspects of human error or the dynamics of teamwork inside the operating room. The occurrence and consequences of process level breakdowns related to inter-team processes and macro-system level communication factors are yet to be addressed with sufficient detail. Additionally, due to the short history of research and limited knowledge in this area, no methods for breakdown detection and management have been developed. Hospitals often implement technology with the intention of improving the quality and safety in surgical patient care. However, during early system design, traditional software development methodologies lack focus on safety concerns. Therefore, new technologies often introduce communication breakdowns, change workflows in inefficient and unintuitive ways and facilitate errors. This book seeks to advance the knowledge on communication and coordination breakdowns in surgical patient care and to develop a breakdown detection method that allows the assessment of the occurrence of breakdowns. In addition, this book seeks to propose a system design framework specific to the communication and coordination requirements of perioperative work such that future socio-technical systems will be designed against breakdown facilitating factors.

This book achieves an in-depth understanding of the impact of breakdowns on surgical work by expanding the focus of analysis beyond teamwork dynamics to include the macro-system communication and coordination processes. The properties of breakdowns and their repairs are studied through the investigation of their occurrence in the operations of two North American surgery units. Through systematic content analysis of breakdown type, theme, tangibility of coordination process employed, coordination scale, breakdown lifetime, repair strategy, and repair cost, several hypotheses derived from previous research findings are tested statistically. The findings reveal that properties of breakdowns determine properties of repairs and that the majority of breakdowns in everyday perioperative work are outside the scope of teamwork – they lie at the inter-team coordination level, i.e. at communication interfaces between micro-systems. Breakdowns are found to propagate downstream in the surgical system. These breakdowns affect the work of multiple teams, which results in increased communication costs associated with the respective repair. Finally, safety is found to relate to the presence or absence of formalized communication structures for re-coordination upon breakdowns. The theoretical implications are materialized into two conceptual models of breakdowns and safety in perioperative work.

In the practical realm, this book offers a breakdown detection method as a useful first step in the management of breakdowns in inter-team coordination within the context of the daily operations of surgical units. To design processes and technology that facilitate coordination and prevent breakdowns, it is necessary that breakdowns are reliably detected and analyzed with respect to their impact on perioperative operations. By mapping information flow expectations for various information needs in clinical work – such as patient status, schedule status, staffing coordination, etc. – a set of predictions can be derived that serves as input to the algorithm for breakdown detection. Evidence is presented for excellent detection performance. The method can be utilized to assess the amount of breakdowns before and after process or technology (re-)design. Additionally, research-based design guidelines and a system design framework are developed.

This book contributes to the knowledge on communication and coordination breakdowns in surgical work as latent conditions having the potential to threaten patient safety. This research provides an initial understanding of the deep features of breakdowns from a process-oriented perspective. From this knowledge, the groundwork for the theoretical models of breakdowns and safety in perioperative activities is built. This book also contributes to the medical operations and systems engineering/informatics communities in two ways. First, by addressing the problem of breakdown management in perioperative work through the breakdown detection method. Second, the practical design guidelines along with the system design framework are proposed based on the novel understanding of breakdowns. In this way, early design activities are tailored to the specific requirements of the domain and consequently prevent breakdowns from occurring or mitigate their impact. Although the detection method and design framework are developed for the surgical space, they can later be extended to cover other clinical and healthcare areas.

Contents

1 Introduction

This book seeks to improve the theoretical and practical knowledge on the management of coordination breakdowns in surgical patient care. The first chapter gives a brief and general introduction into the research reported in this book. It introduces the reader to the domain of surgical patient care, identifies the research problem and challenges, describes the scope of the book and summarizes the theoretical and practical contributions.

Healthcare is defined as the prevention, treatment, and management of illness and the preservation of mental and physical well-being through the services offered by the medical and allied health professions [14]. However, growing numbers of research studies in the past twenty years reveal a reality contradicting this description – around the world, patients become subject to preventable health complications that sometime lead to death of the patient. As many as 98,000 preventable deaths occur per year in the U.S. [41, 157], up to 23,000 in Canada [27], and 850,000 incidents occur in the U.K. [88]. The growing recognition of the frequency and magnitude of avoidable adverse events in healthcare has recently given rise to the field of patient safety. The goal of the patient safety field is the avoidance and prevention of patient injuries or adverse events resulting from the processes of healthcare delivery [261, 285].

As a new discipline, patient safety draws on a significant body of knowledge and expertise from various domains to isolate the causes of adverse events and medical errors, and to develop improvements. Patient safety research methods come from cognitive psychology, engineering, human factors engineering, and organizational management science [86]. The result of a multidisciplinary approach in patient safety is a shift from the search for a single cause to a systems engineering design framework. This type of systems framework seeks to identify all conditions beyond the immediately visible factors that lead to the occurrence of an adverse event. One widely accepted perspective in the analysis of accidents is the idea of active errors and latent factors [238]. Active errors are the directly observable actions resulting in error, occurring at the interaction between a human and some aspect of the socio-technical system – *e.g.* when a medical technician presses the wrong button. Latent factors are less apparent conditions in the socio-technical system that create conditions for error, such as the design of a safety-critical button in a green color, which is conventionally used to signify safe actions. Latent errors are upstream flaws in the design of systems, organizations, management, training, and equipment that lead individuals to make mistakes [86]. Active errors are therefore seen as manifestations of a flawed socio-technical system design.

Research conducted through the trans-disciplinary framework of patient safety identified poor or failed communication between providers of care as one of the most prevalent latent factors across settings that contributes to adverse events [157, 226]. In fact, communication between care providers has consistently remained the main root cause of sentinel events between 1995-2005 [19]. Further, the surgical environment has been found to be the leading sector where such communication problems occur [45, 108, 157].

1.1 Overview of the surgical process

The perioperative process is commonly divided into three stages: pre-operative, operative, and post-operative. During the pre-operative stage, a patient sees a physician in order to diagnose the cause of a particular health concern. During this stage, routine and diagnostic testing is performed, the surgery is scheduled, the patient is educated on her diagnosis and condition, and she is generally prepared for the surgery and the discharge thereafter. The pre-operative stage is distant in time from the day of surgery, except in emergency and trauma cases. The operative stage includes all patient care activities during the day of the surgery and until the surgical procedure is completed – registering and preparing the patient, assessing the state of the patient, assuring the identity of the patient, administering medication, anesthetizing the patient, operating on the patient, planning the continuing care for the patient, etc. In the final post-operative stage, the patient is cared for from the moment the surgical procedure is complete and throughout recovery from surgery until discharge from the hospital. The post-operative stage can span from several hours of post-surgery patient care to several days or weeks. This care includes monitoring the patient state, managing the pain experienced by the patient, and eventually discharging the patient from the hospital. Figure 1 illustrates the three phases of the perioperative process along with the micro-system entities involved at each stage of the surgical patient care.

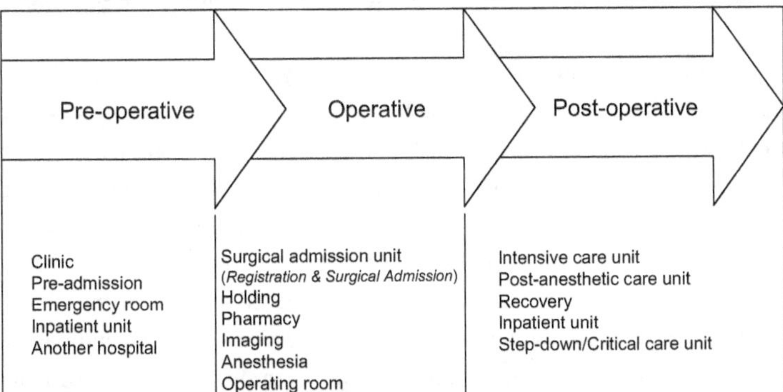

Figure 1: Perioperative process.

As Figure 1 shows, a great number of teams coordinate throughout the continuum of surgical patient care in order to conduct a surgical procedure. The overall perioperative process, comprising all teams and operative stages, is referred to as the surgical macro-system (or just *system*). The surgical care team entities – such as the Pre-admission, Holding or Operating Room (OR) teams –

are micro-systems making up the macro-system. The micro-systems operate individually and synchronously, but are dependent on each other. The macro-system is very complex as it requires the integration of a variety of materials, information, inter-professional work and a flow of inputs from one micro-system to another. Clinicians from several disciplines, along with administrative and support staff must partner, share information, and integrate their efforts. A single patient may be treated by five or more nurses, two or more physicians, associated pharmacists, radiology technicians, test lab and blood bank staff [147]. In addition, support personnel such as patient transporters, supply staff, administrators and others participate in the provision of care services. A variety of instruments, equipment, medications, products and supplies must be planned and prepared for each of the tens of surgeries performed each day. In addition, surgical staff must coordinate and integrate their work with that of external systems. These systems include: emergency department, trauma centers, critical care units, radiology, labs, recovery units, surgical clinics, and others.

Throughout the process, the patient chart is the main artifact coordinating the medical domain problem space among providers of care – it contains all surgery-related information. The chart is continuously reviewed by staff at each micro-system (*i.e.* process step) for completeness – checklists are utilized during preparation for surgery to indicate missing information or test results, and the electronic hospital system is utilized to retrieve or order missing tests, medication, etc.

Work in the surgical unit is characterized by dynamically changing conditions arising from both internal and external factors. These factors cause disturbances or uncertainties associated with planned patient care. For example, an overfilled post-operative inpatient care unit on a given day would result in cancellations of scheduled surgical operations. Also, surgical cases carry an element of unpredictability – elapsed time for surgery can take longer or shorter than expected, and emergencies can affect the planned care for the day. Such uncertainties bring about the need to re-coordinate plans, actions, and patient care goals. The challenge of re-coordination comes from the complexity of managing the interdependency among the multitude of teams and activities [186].

1.2 Breakdowns

Breakdowns in communication and coordination are situations of mismatch between actual and expected conditions in collaborative work. As such, breakdowns present an obstacle to the successful completion of an activity that leads to shift of focus from routine practice to problem solving [121]. Breakdowns are caused by failures in information exchange during the utilization of tools, coordination mechanisms, and cognitive processes. The root causes go beyond the individuals involved – it is the combination of people and the factors in their environment, the socio-technical macro-system level information transfer (i.e. between micro-systems in an organization), that contribute to the instantiation of breakdowns.

Communication breakdowns result in surgery on the wrong patient, the wrong side of the patient, the wrong body part, the wrong implant or the wrong procedure. How can such serious harm occur? One reason for communication failure that has resulted in such harmful effects is when more than one surgeon is involved in the case, such as when the patient care is transferred from one surgeon to another [63]. A different scenario resulting in the wrong patient surgery is linked to mis-communication of patient identity during information handoff between various teams. In one case this involved a total of four teams, including oncology floor, telemetry, neurosurgery, cardiac electrophysiology, and the patient herself [52].

Due to the highly safety-critical nature of surgical operations, breakdowns have the potential for serious patient consequences, as described above. This is not to say that each breakdown necessarily results in harm. There were numerous situations observed in this research when similar breakdowns of miscommunication between teams were detected and patients were not harmed. However, the point of breakdown detection was very close to the door of the OR, *i.e.* to the time when the patient would have been operated on with the wrong assumptions in place. In addition to endangering patient safety, communication breakdowns introduce additional coordination load to an already busy environment. Thus, they are also sources of inefficiency. Although breakdowns do not always manifest themselves as fatal patient outcomes, their persisting occurrence demands further investigation of the latent factors behind them and the prospects of breakdown management in perioperative work.

The patient safety theoretical framework, concerned with events and conditions in the entire system, provides the most appropriate means for breakdown investigation. However, so far, despite the theoretical underpinnings of the discipline, the ultimate locus of patient safety in practice has been the micro-system [86]. Specifically, the immediate environment where care occurs – the operating room, the emergency room, etc. This focus results from the adoption of the systems perspective with a human-centered focus. However, the types of breakdowns described above stem from a higher level of the macro-system and would require not only a human-centered approach of analysis and improvement design, but also a macro process-oriented one.

The research reported in this book includes three studies of the surgical patient care processes in two large teaching hospitals. The book aims to advance the knowledge on communication and coordination breakdowns from the perspective of patient safety. Thus, a multidisciplinary approach is adopted. In addition, the focus of empirical study and analysis is on both the micro- and macro-system levels. Further, this book seeks to develop methodologies for breakdown management through efficient and effective detection. This book is concerned with the macro-management of breakdowns – management through process and system design. This research strives to provide specific surgical environment input to methodologies for the design of processes and technologies, so that the particular requirements of the domain are addressed early in the design cycle.

Note: In this book, although it is recognized that communication is the tool that enables coordination, no explicit distinction between communication and coordination breakdowns is made due to their inherent dependence on one another. Therefore, any reference to breakdowns in this book concerns a breakdown of coordination, which by definition is also one of communication. A more fine-grained view of breakdowns that distinguishes between those of communication and those of coordination is offered in Chapter 6 as a future perspective for fine-grained analysis in the Section "Breakdowns analysis guidelines".

In addition, any reference to 'safety' is intended to refer to patient safety.

1.3 The role of technology

Electronic systems in hospitals facilitate diagnosis, provide channels for communication, and allow data acquisition, processing, storage and sharing. These systems serve as representational systems, decision support systems, communication mediums, coordination tools and information resources. As such, technologies mediate many of the communication and coordination mechanisms in hospital work. In the perioperative setting, technology is used not only in computer-assisted surgery, image-guided surgery, augmented reality surgery, and tele-surgery, but also for patient scheduling, patient record management, patient monitoring, and patient status communication.

When technology is not designed to meet all the requirements of the target domain, *e.g.* of surgical patient care, it can become the trigger of user errors that have disastrous consequences. In fact, evidence from the last two decades reveals that medical devices are so poorly designed and difficult to use that they invite a variety of human errors [26, 160, 210, 318]. Data collected from the U.S. Food and Drug Administration (FDA) between 1985 and 1989 shows that 45–50% of all device recalls stemmed from poor product design [7, 251]. A study also found that 41% of technology interface problems, *i.e.* usability problems, were associated with a subsequent error [163].

The need to address issues of design has prompted a push towards human-centered approaches in technology implementations. In recent years, clinical technology has benefited from several standards. The FDA has revised its Good Manufacturing Practice regulations to include specific requirements for product usability [7]. Guidelines for interface design and usability testing have been published [251] as well as an educational article that specifically covers usability issues [3]. More recent standards for the design of medical devices and technology have also addressed the issues of usability and safety by mandating extensive requirements gathering and the use of usability and human-factors oriented approaches in the development of any device to be used in hospitals (ISO/IEC 62366:2007 [16], ANSI/AAMI-74: 2001 [9], ANSI/AAMI-75:2009 [18], ANSI/AAMI48:1993 [2] and [91, 92]). Most recently, the Agency for Healthcare Research and Quality (AHRQ) recommended that usability become part of the certification test for electronic health records (EHRs) to ensure safety and effectiveness of system integration [19].

The efforts outlined above produced a positive impact on the usability of newly designed systems. Nevertheless, use-errors continue to occur during technology integration. For example, a recent hospital study reported that technology use facilitated 22 previously unexplored error types [160]. These errors fell into two major categories: (1) information errors generated by fragmentation of data and failure to integrate the hospital's several computer and information systems and (2) human-machine interface flaws reflecting machine rules that do not correspond to work organization or usual behaviors. Some of the consequences included dose information problems, conflicting or duplicate medication orders, wrong patient selection, wrong medication selection, loss of data, etc. Another recent study reported that 88% of 176 hospitals experienced serious workflow issues as a result of mismatches between the newly integrated clinical information system and the workflow, which included process and procedure issues, human computer interaction issues, and situation awareness issues [26]. Further, 84% of the hospitals reported critical communication issues that arose from the introduction of a clinical information system as the system changed communication patterns among care providers and departments, and effected inadequate communication between people.

Design that triggers erroneous actions is a communication breakdown at the human-computer interface. The breakdown stems from failed information exchange as a result of the information representation design embedded in the technology interface. The information representation conflicts with the expectation of the human for information representation. The breakdown can also occur at the human-human interface as a result of a conflict between the actual and expected role and function of technology, such as in the case when workflow, process, procedure and communication problems occur as a result of technology integration. Given the evidence of continued design flaws triggering integration problems, a relevant question is: in addition to a user-centered framework, what else can technology design for the surgical setting benefit from? The design of technology could benefit from knowledge on breakdown management.

One explanation for the continued problems of technology integration is that the approaches underpinning the design standards used are generic ergonomics and usability methods, which address the human-cognitive domain of human error in technology use. However, these methods do not account for some critical macro-system requirements of surgical, and clinical, work. The methods are user-centered but not process-oriented. They are focused on the micro-system of direct end-users and neglect the impact that the technology integration will have on other socio-technical micro-systems that interact with the end-user population in providing care for surgical patients. Therefore, an integration of the user-centered and systems perspectives, with a focus on both people and the macro-system processes seems necessary.

The discussion above demonstrates an urgent need to improve safety in the surgical process, as well as in other clinical sectors, at the technology design level – i.e. before accidents occur. So far, there are no design methods specific to the surgical domain. This book delineates the shortcomings of current design practice for clinical systems (Chapter 2), defines requirements for task and workflow modeling with regard to the special characteristics of surgical care, and derives guidelines and a framework for design tailored to the perioperative domain (Chapter 6) that help anticipate and defend against potential breakdowns during the early system design stages.

1.4 Research questions

This book examines the problem of communication and coordination breakdowns and its relevance to surgical operations and safety. Further, the book looks at the potential for prevention of coordination breakdowns through the design of processes and/or technology. The main research question is:

How can we improve surgical care coordination through the informed design of processes and technology that address the specific requirements of perioperative work and consequently prevents or mitigates the occurrence of breakdowns?

To answer this question, the following three sub-questions are addressed:

- **Breakdowns – what are they, really?** Research accounts describe breakdowns as common place in surgical operations. However, knowledge about breakdowns has so far been framed in a narrative qualitative fashion. To manage breakdowns, a deeper understanding of their components and underlying mechanisms is necessary to aid in breakdown solution design. To that end, one must know: What are the properties of breakdowns and coordination mechanisms behind them? What are the relationships among those properties?
- **How can breakdowns be detected and measured?** After acquiring an understanding of breakdowns, the first step towards their management is the ability to detect breakdowns in a formal and systematic way. The ability to detect breakdowns provides a meaningful way to design solutions and evaluate improvement interventions.
- **How can processes and technology be designed to prevent breakdown occurrence?** In designing surgical care systems with the intent to manage coordination and prevent breakdowns associated with integration, it is critical to utilize all the available knowledge about breakdowns in perioperative work. A need exists for integration of domain knowledge about breakdowns (*e.g.* their properties) and design methodology.

1.5 Contributions

The study reported in this book is a first step in the quest to systematically address the occurrence and management of breakdowns, with mixed research methodologies – the study examines the deep features of coordination breakdowns at the surgical macro-system level, addressing inter-team coordination, communication cost, repair strategies and the latent potential of such breakdowns to affect safety. Further, this book offers a method for the detection of breakdowns and a framework for process and technology design tailored to the perioperative domain. The contributions of this book fall into two broad categories within the field of surgical socio-technical system design: theoretical and practical.

1.5.1 Theoretical relevance

As stated earlier in this chapter, in order to improve safety and efficiency in the surgical patient care operations, a need exists for a better understanding of breakdowns in daily clinical work and their latent potential to affect patient safety. This book makes four main contributions to the research in the theoretical space.

- **Mixed methods research design:** This research combines qualitative and quantitative techniques in the examination of problems that were previously addressed only qualitatively. In particular, in addition to the qualitative observation and analysis, breakdowns are coded based on particular properties derived from existing theory and research, and statistical relationships of dependence among those properties is established (Chapter 3).
- **Understanding of breakdowns:** As a result of the mixed methods research design approach, a novel and detailed understanding of the deep features of breakdowns is acquired (Chapter 4 and [269, 270, 272]). Breakdown properties are found to determine repair properties, including the communication overhead, the number of interruptions, and the safety threats incurred by a breakdown. Such in-depth understanding of the underlying mechanisms of coordination, breakdowns and safety, based on quantitative statistical evidence, is new and a major step towards the management of breakdowns in surgical operations.

  In the area of technology adoption, this book offers an incremental contribution by identifying a systemic culture problem – the issue of trust among patient care teams – as a disabler to successful technology adoption.
- **Conceptual model of breakdowns in the surgical process:** A theoretical model of breakdowns is proposed that integrates the knowledge acquired through this research with previous coordination models from organizational science (Chapter 4 and [270]). The result is a conceptual model of breakdowns specific to the surgical process. The model can be utilized in the detection and analysis of breakdowns, and in system design.
- **Conceptual model of safety and breakdowns:** Based on the findings of this study, this book suggests a conceptual model of safety and breakdowns (Chapter 4). In particular, the model reflects a relationship between the existence or absence of formal re-coordination mechanisms upon a breakdown and the potential that the breakdown will affect safety.

1.5.2 Practical relevance

The knowledge acquired through the empirical study presented in this book is the foundation for addressing the practical problems of breakdown management through process and technology design (*i.e.* system design) in the perioperative setting. To that end, this book makes two major contributions.

- **Breakdown detection method:** This book offers a method for the detection of breakdowns – automated or manual, inspired by both the insights acquired through this research and the approaches to breakdown detection in other computational and social sciences (Chapter 5 and [274]). The proposed detection method is validated through its application over the data collected from both hospitals studied in this research.
- **Framework for process/technology design:** To aid the management of breakdowns in the surgical setting, this book develops a set of guidelines based on the newly acquired understanding of breakdowns. A design framework is proposed that integrates the guidelines with strategies adopted in other industries. The framework targets system (re-)design that supports coordination in surgical patient care by preventing and avoiding breakdowns from occurring (Chapter 6 and [270, 271, 273]).

1.6 Outline

Chapter 2 provides a review of the literature on patient safety and medical error in healthcare, and introduces the problem of communication and coordination breakdowns within surgical operations. In addition, the methodologies used in medical technology design and their shortcomings to meet the requirements for support of surgical work are presented. The novel aspects introduced by this book are highlighted throughout the topics. The chapter concludes with a formulation of the problem statement, a framework for this research that derives a set of properties to be explored in the formal analysis of breakdowns, and a set of hypotheses to be examined.

Chapter 3 presents this research's design to the study of breakdowns in the perioperative unit. The choice for research methodology is justified and the two surgical units are described. The coding scheme to aid in the categorization of observational data for purposes of quantitative analysis is developed and the measurements of breakdown properties are defined. The longitudinal study of technology adoption, examining coordination breakdowns occurrence prior and post- integration of an electronic whiteboard communication tool in the surgical unit is described as well.

Chapter 4 integrates all the findings from this research into three main categories: qualitative, quantitative and technology adoption-related outcomes. Significant relationships between breakdown properties and resulting repair properties are identified. The findings indicate a complex interplay between process workflow, coordination theme, breakdown lifetime, repair strategies and cost. The implications are discussed and the chapter concludes with an abstraction of the findings into two theoretical models: one of breakdowns in the surgical process, and the other of the relationship of breakdowns to safety.

Chapter 5 presents a method for breakdown detection in the perioperative context inspired by computational approaches concerned with breakdown detection in other domains. Following a brief review of the relevant literature, the breakdown detection method targeting the surgical process is developed. An extensive evaluation is provided through the application of the method over the data collected from both surgical units.

Chapter 6 focuses on the practical implications of the insights gained through this research in terms of breakdown management through process improvement and through technology. The chapter begins by materializing this study's findings into specific guidelines for analysis and design of processes and technology for the surgical setting. The chapter concludes with a discussion of the directions for future work in breakdown management in the perioperative setting.

Chapter 7 concludes the book with a summary of the major findings, key contributions, and perspectives for future work.

2

Communication and breakdowns in the domain of surgery – related work and book hypotheses

Breakdowns in communication and coordination in surgical work have the potential for disastrous consequences. This chapter describes the complexity of coordination demand in surgical patient care, the magnitude of the problem of adverse events, and the approaches to understanding the causes behind breakdown sentinel events. A review of previous research on communication and coordination breakdowns in perioperative work is offered, which is then used to formulate the framework and hypotheses for the study of breakdowns presented in this book. The role of technology design and processes are also examined and shortcomings of current system design methods for clinical technology are analyzed. The identification of shortcomings reveals potential for improvement of systems design at the methodological level.

Patient safety is of utmost importance to healthcare providers, consumers and technology manufacturers. However, evidence demonstrates that there is a risk for the patient associated with every admission to a hospital – a risk that is independent of a medical condition and stems from human and systemic factors [144, 157]. Communication breakdowns, in particular, are a major cause of hospital adverse events [108, 157, 171, 226, 299]. Breakdowns result in longer length of patient stay, increased patient anxiety, tension among staff, increased resource use, loss of revenue, staff dissatisfaction, and a decrease in the quality and safety of patient care, including a high percentage of adverse events [178, 233, 243, 246, 317]. Consequently, recent research on healthcare improvement has focused on the systems and socio-technical issues in patient care. To that end, a multi-level approach to change has been recommended that includes the individual, group/team and organizational levels, as well as the larger professional, social and organizational context in the care continuum [93, 109]. At all levels, the role of information technology is critical as well.

Information technology plays an essential role in the coordination of perioperative work – both in the medical problem space and in the clinical activity space. Information systems facilitate diagnosis (*e.g.* decision-support systems), provide channels for communication (*e.g.* electronic patient record systems), tools for coordination of patient care (*e.g.* patient scheduling systems), and allow data acquisition, processing, storage and sharing. As such, technologies mediate many processes in hospital work. Their role in clinical care has, however, been shown to have negative consequences. A great number of adverse events have been triggered by poorly designed technology [1, 48, 157] and breakdowns have been introduced into clinical work as the result of technology introduction into the workflow [26, 160]. When technology is not designed with the user in mind, it may facilitate the administration of a lethal dose of radiation [48] or chemotherapeutic agent [1]. Many patients have died and medical professionals lost their professional standing as a result of inadequate system design [41]. The issues of human-computer interaction, cognition, and usability have become essential to the design of healthcare technology. Alas, the generic methods proposed by these domains do not completely cover the critical requirements of safety-critical clinical work and no design methodologies specific to the clinical domain have been developed.

Given the pressing need for improvement of communication in the provision of surgical patient care, this research investigates the occurrence of breakdowns at a novel depth – through the examination of their properties and their relationship to coordination mechanisms in surgical processes. Further, the book examines how the newly acquired knowledge about breakdowns can inform the design of processes and information technology so as to prevent future breakdowns in perioperative work. The present chapter provides a review of the literature on patient safety and medical error in healthcare, and introduces the research on the problem of communication and coordination breakdowns within surgical operations. In addition, the methodologies used in medical technology design, and their shortcomings to meet the requirements for support of surgical work, are presented. The novel aspects introduced by this book are highlighted throughout the topics. Finally, the chapter develops a formulation of the framework for this research and the hypotheses to be examined through it.

Due to the multidisciplinary nature of work in the field of patient safety, the literature on the topic of communication and coordination breakdowns, as well as on computer-mediated clinical work comes from a variety of publishing venues – medical, nursing, social science, medical informatics, computer science, and systems engineering journals and conferences, as well as national and international governmental bodies' publications. In the review of the literature presented in this chapter and in the rest of the book, the following sources were searched for articles published up to July 2010:

- Scientific digital libraries: ScienceDirect, ACM, IEEE, PubMed, Patient Safety Network (PSNet)
- Government bodies: The Food and Drug Administration (FDA), Agency for Healthcare Research and Quality (AHRQ), International Standards Organization (ISO), Institute for Safe Medication Practices (ISMP), Association for the Advancement of Medical Instrumentation (AAMI), National Health Service (NHS), World Health Organization (WHO), Institute for Healthcare Improvement (IHI), Institute of Medicine (IOM)
- Google scholar: combinations of the search terms "communication, breakdowns, surgical, OR, surgery"
- Three special issues of the Cognition, Technology & Work journal were reviewed: one on enhancing surgical systems [125], another on large-scale coordination in healthcare [207], and the third on ethnographic research in healthcare [310].

The resulting review of the literature spans publications from each of the scientific areas listed above.

2.1 Patient safety and the significance of adverse events

The publication of the Institute of Medicine's report "To Err is Human" in 1999 [157] was one of the first to expose the severity and frequency of occurrence of preventable errors in hospitals due to human factors and systemic design issues – reporting that as many as 98,000 people die per year in the U.S. from adverse events. Similar studies with equally alarming findings were conducted in other nations – the U.K. [88], Canada [27], and Australia [300]. Data collected from the Physician Insurers Association of America between 1985 and 2003 revealed that 70% of medical errors come from the hospital setting [11]. Research on the frequency of adverse events in hospitals followed. A study of 51 hospitals in the U.S. found that adverse events occurred in 3.7% of patient admissions [44]. Another investigation, involving 28 Australian hospitals, revealed a 16.6% adverse event rate [300], where the complications resulted in patient death in a total of 4.9% of hospitalized patients. A research study in the U.K. reported a 10.8% adverse event rate, with 8% of all adverse events being fatal [286]. A different study, in the U.S., warned that each day spent in a hospital increased the likelihood of experiencing an adverse event by 6% [23]. A systematic review of the literature on in-hospital adverse events concluded that the median overall incidence of preventable complications was 9.2% - one in every ten patients, where 7.4% of adverse events were lethal [74]. The cost of adverse events was estimated at $4700 per preventable event in an American hospital [35]. These studies led to a considerable rise in patient safety research and funding, and the shift in focus from causes of clinical malpractice to organizational socio-technical factors [265].

2.1.1 Adverse events and the surgical setting

Between 39.6% and 48% of medical errors in a hospital come from surgical operations [11, 23, 27]. Wrong site surgery is a very common example of an adverse surgical event [51]. The term describes an incident resulting from procedures performed on the wrong patient, the wrong body part, or the wrong body site. It also applies to cases when the wrong procedure, an unnecessary or unauthorized procedure, is performed. Another common example is related to medication administration – the wrong medication or the wrong dosage may be administered, or the medication may be given to the wrong patient [1, 48]. These types of adverse events occur across hospital settings – inpatient or ambulatory, emergency room or intensive care surgical settings. While multiple factors usually contribute to an accident of this type, the most common reason behind wrong site surgery and medication errors is communication breakdown [15, 226]. These breakdowns derive either from inter-personal communication or are facilitated by communication via coordinating artifacts such as paper forms, electronic records, or medical device interfaces.

As outlined above, issues of communication in perioperative work are a serious source of harm to patients, in addition to exhausting already strained healthcare resources. This book seeks to address precisely the problem of understanding and managing communication breakdowns with the intent to improve safety, work conditions, and operational efficiency.

2.1.2 Understanding the causes of adverse events

"Human error in medicine, and the adverse events that may follow, are problems of psychology and engineering, not of medicine." – John Senders, 1993

Prior to the rise of the field of patient safety, adverse events were examined in the light of personal accountability and malpractice with a primary focus on active errors – those proximal actions that directly led to an incident. Through the emerging discipline of patient safety, a wide recognition that recurring types of medical error transcend specific organizations and settings was established. This realization set out the conditions for more comprehensive research into the underlying factors of adverse events. Thus, critical assumptions about errors in healthcare evolved from a focus on a single cause, legalistic framework to a systems engineering design framework [86] that integrates approaches from cognitive psychology, engineering, human factors, and organizational management science. The adoption of systems engineering approaches in the manufacturing, logistics, distribution, aviation, and transportation industries had produced a significant positive impact. Still, the application of systems engineering to the domain of healthcare has been slow to rise. Efforts to advocate the integration of the two started in the 1990s [157, 171] and continue today – a recent joint report from the National Academy of Engineering and the Institute of Medicine called for widespread application of systems engineering tools to improve healthcare [12].

The systems engineering perspective framework defines an engineering process of identifying a system of interest, choosing appropriate performance measures, selecting a modeling tool, studying model properties and behavior under a variety of scenarios, and making design and operational decisions for implementation [159]. The notion of a system reflects a set of diverse entities, or micro-systems – such as nurses, physicians, functional units, etc. Systems engineering sets the focus of analysis on coordination, synchronization, and integration of complex systems of people, information, artifacts, and financial resources [161]. The key property of safety is defined as one that emerges from the proper interaction of micro-systems of the healthcare system (National Patient Safety Foundation [64]). The interaction of the micro-systems as they execute their functions gives rise to a global system behavior. A system is also characterized by a state in relation to preconditions and time, and through the system's operation the state changes. The state traces (*i.e.* history) can be used to compute performance measures. The system is modeled by identifying and representing the most relevant system characteristics through a variety of techniques – *e.g.* a process model, human factors model, statistical model, stochastic process model, etc., in order to analyze the system behavior and improve it.

The motivation to apply systems engineering to healthcare is to reduce errors by redesigning systems and processes using human factors principles, with special attention to tools, technology, organizations and people [86]. As a consequence of the shift to systems thinking, the causes of incidents in healthcare are now recognized as system properties that often remain hidden and invisible until an adverse event occurs [219]. The strength of the systems approach is that it exposes latent factors – upstream defects embedded in the system design – through intensive system evaluation, while discounting active errors caused by human beings [239, 240]. Investigative techniques and trans-disciplinary analysis of both latent and active errors as threats to the system facilitate the application of the systemic framework [128].

The most influential conceptual model used in systems reliability science and in the analysis of healthcare adverse events is known as the Swiss Cheese Model [238]. It encapsulates the idea that an organization's design is layered with defenses, barriers, and safeguards to protect the safety of the system. The assumption is that each defense layer (*i.e.* cheese slice) has multiple design weaknesses, similar to holes in the Swiss cheese slices. The presence of these weaknesses does not necessarily make the system unsafe at any one time, but rather only when the holes in all layers momentarily align to permit a trajectory of accident opportunity. The holes in the defenses arise for two reasons – active failures and latent conditions [239]. The former are the unsafe acts committed by people who are in direct contact with the patient or system. The latter arise as a direct consequence of faulty decisions by management, designers, builders, and procedure writers. Latent conditions can lie dormant until they align with local antecedent conditions to create an unsafe system state. The model is illustrated in Figure 2a.

To understand organizational system accidents, it is suggested that the interaction of active and latent failures must be examined in the light of organizational processes, task and environment antecedents, individual unsafe acts and failed defenses (Figure 2b). Performance influencing factors and error producing conditions such as high workload, poor supervision or training (*i.e.* latent factors) can influence actions in a way to facilitate active errors such as slips, lapses, or mistakes. Violations of safe practices, protocols and standards (*i.e.*

active errors) are also seen as the outcomes of low organizational morale and issues in management (*i.e.* latent factors). At the core of the Swiss cheese model is the notion that behind each adverse event are a series of latent factors distant from the time and site of the adverse event.

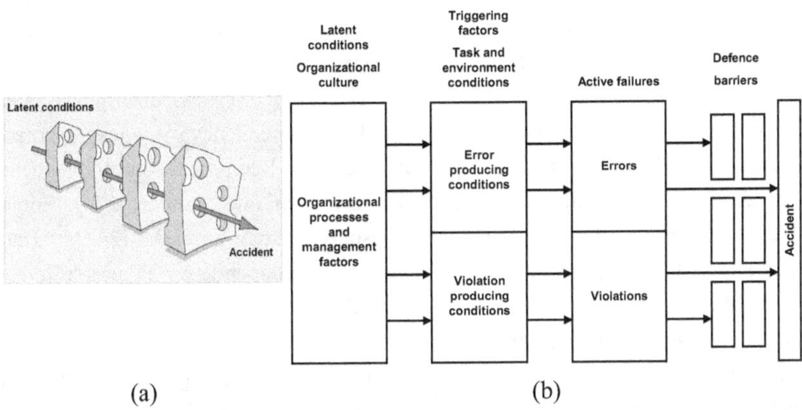

(a) (b)

Figure 2a: The Swiss cheese model (Reproduced from [239]). Figure 2b: The Swiss cheese model as an organizational accident causation model for medical accidents (Reproduced from [241]).

The Swiss cheese perspective provides the foundation for the study of latent conditions in surgical environments, such as communication breakdowns. Patient safety advocates indicate a need to focus more on latent failures and less on active ones [136, 144, 157]. This book is focused on the study of such latent communication failures. While the Swiss cheese model is not the leading framework of analysis for this work, it is presented here to provide the background understanding of the construct of latent failures that defines the nature of the breakdowns under investigation. This work uses the systems engineering framework to acquire a novel understanding of communication and coordination breakdowns – critical latent factors that have been identified in previous research of perioperative systems as a major cause of preventable incidents – through a detailed and thorough analysis of their occurrence.

2.2 Communication and coordination in clinical work

In healthcare, coordination is highly complex – a reflection of the complexity and the magnitude of the healthcare system. In theoretical terms, clinical services are joint activities that involve a number of agents (*e.g.* physician, nurse, technologist, pharmacist, etc.) who work towards a common goal of providing healthcare. Clinical activity is not only a highly cooperative process, but also safety-critical, distributed over time and space, and characterized by high coordination demand. Coordination bonds participants' actions into a coherent joint activity [54]. Communication enables coordination, which in turn facilitates the cooperation processes [54, 156]. Communication and coordination mechanisms are direct or mediated by information technologies.

Coordination is determined by several distinct types of micro-system dependencies. Along a workflow, sequential interdependency manages the correct sequences of tasks among multiple teams. Reciprocal interdependence characterizes the mutual dependency of teams on one another [279]. Pooled interdependency refers to the shared resources among teams [243]. "Team arrangement" reflects the effect of intensified interdependency as an additive of sequential, reciprocal and pooled, to produce higher levels of coordination demand [280]. Team arrangement is best representative of the degree of interdependency that coordination in healthcare must manage. The quality and efficiency of care is a function of the successful management of the high-bandwidth interdependency [106]. In fact, the Association of Operating Room Nurses (AORN) lists coordination of care for surgical patients as the first item in the outline of the responsibilities of perioperative nursing practice. AORN specifies communication skills as a key component of coordination [202].

In practical terms, the complexity comes from the large number of groups, or micro-systems that must coordinate their individual efforts for the administration of effective patient care. In addition, coordination is problematic because multiple experts must make dynamic decisions based on the patient history and evolution of the patient's state. Hospitals provide procedures and processes for coordination, which sometimes fail, for various reasons – e.g. exceptional cases, non-transmission of information, non-compliance, and others [213]. A delay or blockage in one part of the patient care journey will have a ripple effect resulting in delays throughout the continuum of care. As a result, coordination of activities relies heavily on mutual adjustment to address contingencies [186]. The fragmentation in the healthcare system also increases the coordination demand as the process requires documentation to be duplicated between departments and disciplines because of the lack of integration of information tools among providers [133].

In order to better understand the sources of complexity and the challenges of coordination in hospital environments, several researchers set out to study the patterns of communication and coordination that define current clinical practice.

Observational studies reported that clinicians have a preference for direct synchronous – face-to-face or phone – communication [57, 65, 66]. This phenomenon reflects the urgency in trying to acquire critical information when it is not available. A study on information-seeking behaviors also found that the predominant reason for seeking information of all types was direct patient care [65]. Further, communication and coordination were observed to occur most often in an informal fashion – through conversation, observation, or informal paper documentation (*e.g.* notes) [57, 119, 230, 313].

Coiera's work examined communication and information access patterns in hospital work. Coiera's research employed semi-structured interviews, observations of 12 clinical workers performing routine duties, and the thematic extraction of emerging patterns [57]. The author noted that communication problems occurred more frequently than information access problems and that the environment was highly interrupt-driven. Frequent opportunistic interruptions by face-to-face communications were driven by a need for acknowledgement of receipt of the message communicated. Consequently, the work plans of workers were constantly rescheduled and tasks were postponed because there seemed to be pressure to deal with events when they arose. In a different study, Coiera looked at communication traffic through the observation of 8 physicians and 2 nurses [58]. What he found was that medical staff generated twice as many outgoing communication events as they received. Outgoing calls were directed to booking and other medical and administrative staff. Conversations with medical colleagues (42% of call traffic) were regarding specific patient details, diagnosis and therapy. Coiera reported that many tasks involved a series of phone calls, some of them tracking contact information for functional roles. Due to the high phone traffic, clinicians utilized a convention to judge the urgency of an incoming call from the call origin as well as the number of successive incoming calls. Based on these studies, the author recommended using wireless technology to address mobility issues, a message board with some form of acknowledgement mechanism for tasks, a role-based database directory, attaching an "urgency" to task requests, improved collaboration among team members, and informal data capture [58]. He further developed these ideas in [59], where he advocates that the importance of informal transactions in clinical work needs to be recognized and supported by system design. In addition, tasks that require grounding between agents should be supported by synchronous communication mediums. Finally, tasks that do not require grounding can be formalized through the use of computational tools such as software.

Other researchers, Xiao et al., sought to acquire knowledge on the communication patterns specific to surgical work. Xiao et al. conducted ethnographic studies in three OR suites and for a total of 100 hours of observations [201, 306]. The researchers coded the data in terms of the duration, mode, recipient of information, and the purpose of communication observed. What the investigation revealed was consistent with Coiera's findings – the majority of communication was synchronous - face to face (70%), by telephone (19%) and through intercom (7%). Communication with clinical staff that are physically distant, or those on a different floor or unit, was predominantly accomplished via the phone. Most observed communications lasted less than one minute (94%) and most were in regards to equipment (38%) and patient preparedness (26%). The communication episodes of longer duration were related to surgical patient scheduling, re-scheduling, room assignment, and staffing. Similar findings were reported from two more of their studies [200, 202], with the notable difference that the main reasons for communication were scheduling and patient preparedness. The authors suggest that automatic tracking of information can greatly decrease communication and interruptions. An electronic representation of patient status, in particular an electronic board, would eliminate a great deal of the communication load of surgical care providers.

In a related study, Xiao et al. defined the critical role of the OR whiteboard, an external coordinating artifact, in the operations of the surgical suite [308]. The whiteboard was a facilitator for coordination negotiation, joint planning and decision making, and it augmented inter-personal communication. As such, the whiteboard alleviated much of the burden of coordination. Additionally, the whiteboard was used in an informal fashion for messaging among clinical staff. The authors conclude that the use of artifacts has a profound impact on coordination processes.

A different strand of work on coordination in healthcare is concerned with coordination in clinical work reliant on implicit mechanisms such as standards, formal and informal rules, and cultural conventions [110, 112]. A surgery, in particular, depends on the collaboration of a number of care providers – surgeons, anesthesiologists, nurses, technicians, the transport team and others. It also depends on the readiness of the OR, the provision of specialized equipment and supplies, the readiness of the patient, etc. These dependencies are critical and implicated at the system level in the design of processes and procedures. Implicit coordination occurs also at the team, or micro-system level. Xiao et al. conducted numerous observations in various trauma OR environments [304, 309]. In the analysis of 17 video recorded trauma resuscitation cases they found several forms of non-communication task coordination activities: following protocols, following the leader's foci and actions, anticipation of the leader's needs, and more generally activity monitoring [304, 309]. The authors recommended that coordination support devices, such as large panel displays and wearable communicators can improve communication by increasing the activity monitoring capabilities of team members.

The frequent utilization of implicit means of coordination has raised concerns regarding safety. The assumption is that implicit coordination, while efficient, predisposes to breakdowns resulting in adverse patient care outcomes. Work in aviation addressed similar safety concerns through major team training efforts in explicit coordination strategies and protocols [297]. This approach, advocated for healthcare as well, can have implications for systems design. While many studies identify coordination-related communication as the root cause of medical errors [157, 226], the literature review found no data on the specific types of coordination that are problematic. One of the goals of this book is to examine coordination processes at a finer level of detail than the high-level concept of coordination thereby identifying specific coordination mechanisms that are associated with breakdowns.

This book integrates the knowledge on communication and coordination patterns in clinical work, presented in this section, into a framework for the analysis of breakdowns. By analyzing breakdowns in terms of the communication and coordination process, one is able to investigate the relationship between the process and the properties of breakdowns. The result is a more formalized and deep understanding of the dependencies between coordination processes and breakdown occurrence than was previously available.

2.3 Breakdowns

Given the complexity, high coordination demand, high workload and high stress that characterize surgical work, it is not surprising that there are opportunities for error and that breakdowns occur. However, the alarming fact is the high incidence rate – the surgical environment is the most common site for adverse events in a hospital, across geographical boundaries, with communication breakdown being the most frequent cause [27, 45, 108, 157, 170]. In fact, Wilson et al. found that in healthcare communication failures were twice as common as errors attributable to inadequate skill [299]. It is also known that the majority of communication breakdown adverse events are related to surgery [27].

Studies such as the ones described above demonstrate the critical roles of communication and information to the safe operation of surgical units. The complexity coupled with the fragmentation of the healthcare system has, however, resulted in significant process inefficiencies that also affect safety. Clinicians spend the majority of their time on information and communication related activities instead of actual patient care. A recent time and motion study of 36 surgical units revealed that nurses spend 35% of their time working on documentation and 21% on care coordination (communication with team members or other departments). Patient care activities accounted for 19% of nurses' work time, and only 7% was on actual patient assessment and reading vital signs. In addition, 6.6% of nurses' time was found to be wasteful, or non-value added – spent on hunting and gathering information. Given the high workload and stress that characterize the environment in which so much effort is spent on documentation and coordination, it is not surprising that the quality of information accuracy and/or exchange is affected.

Breakdowns in communication, verbal or written, can take many forms – miscommunications within a medical practice, communication failures between components of the healthcare system, or between providers of care working different shifts [10]. Further, breakdowns can occur between different healthcare providers, such as between primary care physicians and emergency room personnel, ancilliary services, nursing homes and other patient services in hospitals. Common communication problems are: poorly documented or lost information on lab results, diagnostic testing, medication information, etc. Breakdowns are present in teamwork – between health care professionals working synchronously in one location on the same patient. Breakdowns also affect the communication among multiple care teams distributed in various physical spaces, as well as between healthcare providers and patients. One study reported that a fifth of communication breakdowns involved more than two entities [20]. An example of such coordination breakdown is a misplaced patient. In the process of receiving care, patients are transferred through multiple wards and units – pre-operative holding, emergency department, operating room suite, intensive care unit, etc. These transfer activities force coordination across micro-system boundaries. One study of the intensive care unit reported that in a three year period, eight patients were misplaced within the hospital, four of which were 'lost' during the transfer out of the unit [206]. The patients were later located when the need for care arose. Similar issues with tracking patients have been previously described in the emergency department, clinic, intensive care, rehabilitation and other hospital settings [77, 95, 289].

Dealing with breakdowns in surgery disables the progress of patient care and takes resources away from actual care. A study found that perioperative clinicians spent 12.7% of their highest workload time repairing breakdowns, instead of working towards patient care [269]. Such amount of repair work is excessive given the critical nature of the activities and has direct implications for efficiency, throughput and process cost. In addition, fixing breakdowns adds a layer of complexity to the work, increases the level of uncertainty that needs to be communicated among care providers throughout the surgical system, and creates opportunities for further breakdowns.

Relevant to the issue of communication breakdowns is the notion of information flow. Information should flow accurately and in a timely fashion among providers of care. In reality, information often does not follow the patient upon her transfer from one point of care to another. When information is not available, a communication breakdown has occurred that will delay patient care and present a latent safety-threatening condition. Information flow is critical in making medication prescription decisions, in acquiring test results, and in coordination of medication orders at points of interface or transfer of care [10]. One study found that the most common information flow issues were inadequate dissemination of drug knowledge (29%) and inadequate availability of information about the patient (18%) [171]. Additionally, all errors identified in that study stemmed from impaired access to information. In a different study, physicians reported that their information needs were met only 30% of the time [66]. Many breakdowns were also found to be associated with contactability issues – a clinician was successfully contacted only 74% of the time [58].

The research findings reviewed suggest that successful reduction in communication breakdowns can substantially improve patient safety [108]. There is a consensus that further research on the problem of communication breakdowns needs to be conducted [226]. To that end, a number of endeavors in healthcare have been devoted to the ethnographic study of breakdowns. The majority of such work is focused on the investigation of the behavior of one team/micro-system. Nevertheless, this book will review the teamwork research as it provides some relevant insights. This book will contribute to existing work with expanding the scope and depth of analysis and consequent knowledge on breakdowns in surgical work. Further, the book will propose a method for breakdowns detection to facilitate improvement initiatives and will offer a system design framework informed by the novel understanding of breakdowns.

2.3.1 Breakdowns in OR teamwork

Some of the communication breakdowns in surgical work originate from activity inside the operating room where the surgical team consisting of nurses, surgeons, anesthesiologists, perfusionists, residents and students conducts the surgical procedures. This is one of the critical micro-systems in the perioperative process where team dynamics and communication can directly affect patient safety. The majority of ethnographic research in patient safety in surgery focuses on the study of this micro-system in relative isolation from the rest. The assessments tend to focus on the teamwork performance inside the operating room theatre, at the exclusion of the wider system [125]. This section reviews previous research on breakdowns inside the OR in order to present a comprehensive picture of the state of knowledge on the topic of breakdowns in surgical operations. The relevant recommendations derived in each study are noted as well, if any.

The work of Xiao et al. on OR teams utilized video recordings for the thematic analysis of situations during which breakdowns occurred in 17 OR trauma cases [304, 309]. The researchers found that coordination breakdowns in teamwork happened during crisis situations such as when there is pressure to seek alternative solutions, when an unexpected/non-routine procedure is initiated, and when there is a diffusion of responsibility. The breakdowns stemmed from conflicting plans, inadequate support in crisis situations, inadequate verbalization of problems, and lack of task delegation. Coordination breakdowns occurred often when there was lack of explicit communication. In the study of other surgical settings, Xiao et al. reported that conventions of practice utilized by clinicians in perioperative work were prominent [307]. For example, charge nurses and anesthesiologists balanced the effort required to gather information against the value of accurate information by performing optimal sampling. This suggested that in many cases patient care is performed under situations of incomplete information.

In a related study, Plasters et al. examined the information needs essential to the operations of an OR suite [230]. Through an integration of 24 hours of observational data and a version of the Critical Incident Technique, they found that the major information challenges were related to patient status, patient room location, scheduled surgery, anesthesia staff status, room staff status, equipment status and location, special needs, surgeon disposition and availability, pending changes and staff location and availability. The sources that surgical staff turned to for such information were IT systems, documents, direct observation, and social networks.

Healey et al. conducted observations of 22 laparoscopic surgeries. They measured teamwork performance factors and found that equipment, work environment and procedure contributed to distractions and interruptions [126]. For instance, they observed that surgeons and associated personnel within the sterile zone frequently experienced mid-operation problems related to the ergonomics of the equipment or the setup of the environment. This resulted in frequent movement around the equipment. In addition, breakdowns outside of the OR theatre brought external staff into the operating room, interrupting the work, and sometimes causing dedicated surgical staff to leave the operating room. These interruptions exacerbated the effects of other distracting events. Other sources of interference were beepers, phone calls, and other conversations about matters irrelevant to the case at hand.

The study of Catchpole et al. observed 24 pediatric cardiac surgeries and 20 orthopedic ones, examining the errors that occurred in teamwork [49]. The researchers found several commonalities, despite the differing demands of the two types of surgeries. The most frequent non-technical errors were planning failures & workload management (37%), failures in situation awareness (34-42%), and teamwork and coordination errors (19%). Effective situational diagnosis and real time evaluation during dynamic team work tasks were advised for enhanced performance.

Guerlain and colleagues studied the issue of situation awareness and communication during 10 laparoscopic surgeries [113]. Through a structured questionnaire administered post-surgery, they found that the surgeon was the primary holder of critical patient and case information, while the other team members lacked awareness of important information in regards to the procedure they co-performed with the surgeon. This was due to the fact that no pre-procedural briefings took place. In a follow-up study, the researchers implemented a teamwork intervention to improve communication in the OR [114]. They implemented a Crew Resource Management (CRM) training program (see Appendix D.1) for surgical staff. The program emphasized callouts of key events for situation awareness, read-back of requests for breakdown prevention, and time for voicing concerns and utilizing debriefings following surgeries for continuous learning. Pre-incision briefing protocols were also introduced for the whole OR team – patient history and the objectives for the surgery were reviewed, including contingencies and the possibilities of conversion to different types of procedures. The observations of 40 cases performed with the CRM communication protocol led to the conclusion that the training had an impact on briefing practices for 4 out of the 5 surgeons. Further, the intervention led to increased scores on questionnaire measures of communication and observed situational awareness.

Simlar to the above study, Whyte et al. also investigated the effects of team briefings on the quality of communication in the operating room [294]. Using qualitative analysis of fieldnotes from 302 team briefings, they reported a positive impact. However, they also cautioned to some unintended effects of the implementation of such structured communication: team briefings could mask knowledge gaps, disrupt positive communication, reinforce professional divisions, create tension, and perpetuate a problematic culture of professional divisions. Thus, they concluded that interventions that affect inter-professional teamwork must be sensitive to social and cultural factors of the target setting.

Kountantji et al. implemented a different kind of intervention – a simulation-based communication training program that included briefings and checklists, designed to enhance planning and support workflow [162]. Nine surgical teams were observed during simulations. The study revealed that the training did not appear to greatly improve non-technical skill performance. This finding contrasts with other research such as Guerlain's.

Lingard et al.'s work, based on observations of 48 surgeries and a total of 90 hours, reported that communication failures occurred in 30% of information exchanges [178]. Breakdowns were categorized as being communication of poor timing (46%), missing or inaccurate information (36%), exclusion of key individuals from the communication (21%), and system effect breakdowns – inefficiency, team tension, resource waste, workaround, delay, etc. (37%). One third of breakdowns had the potential to jeopardize patient safety by creating tension, interrupting the routine work, increasing memory load, and inefficiency.

The research of Parush et al. on team communication during open-heart surgeries examined the speech acts of team members in the OR to identify problematic loops of information flow within the team [221]. The authors reported that 49% of situational awareness related communication in the OR was found susceptible to information loss. The findings were used to derive requirements for an augmentative information display to support situation awareness in the operating room of their study.

The strong evidence that communication breakdowns in the OR are commonplace across organizations and around the world prompted the WHO to publish guidelines for safe surgery in 2008 [17]. This effort was followed by a study, conducted by Haynes and colleagues who designed a surgical safety checklist to improve team communication and consistency of care in the OR [124]. The checklist required that the surgical team verbally review all expected critical events and confirm all basic steps during surgery. The study collected data on clinical processes and outcomes before and after the introduction of the checklist in the ORs of hospitals in eight countries around the world. The researchers reported that the checklist reduced the rate of death by half (from 1.5% to 0.8%) and the rate of complications from 11% to 7%. Following Haynes et al.'s report the surgical checklist uptake around the world has been rapid. However, some studies have shown that such checklists are associated with lack of compliance past implementation time [177], which may be a result of socio-organizational factors.

The insights provided by the studies of breakdowns in the OR have advanced the understanding of teamwork in high-risk clinical care and are valuable within the teamwork frame. However, a number of adverse events investigations have identified breakdowns at the macro system level, i.e. between multiple teams/groups/units, as the cause of accidents [1, 52, 56, 157, 226, 276]. Root causes are often positioned at the systemic level - inter-professional communication, organizational culture differences, lack of common standards across settings, etc. The studies on team dynamics confined the focus of analysis of breakdowns to the view of one collocated group, or micro-system – i.e. focusing on intra-team communication processes within the OR. Therefore, the findings related to teamwork processes are insufficient to offer input beyond the teamwork frame – at the macro system level where the issues of micro-system interfaces lye. Additionally, the recommendations proposed were specific solutions and did not extend to the methodological space. There is a need for a better understanding of breakdowns at the systems level. Moreover, we need to understand how breakdowns impact the safety and efficiency of operations. With this knowledge, processes and technology can be (re-)designed for a safer surgical patient care. This book takes a lead in this direction.

2.3.2 Breakdowns at large in perioperative work

Despite the need to improve the quality and safety of surgical patient care at the macro-system level, research on breakdowns at large is scarce. Only lately a shift in focus to the macro-system issues occurred. This shift is marked by several studies. Specifically, ethnographic work reported some coordination breakdowns at group boundaries in the perioperative setting, and their consequences [206, 243]. These studies denote an important turn to the proactive investigation of latent factors at the macro-system level, with a focus on inter-team processes. It was these types of healthcare system factors that were commonly the output of earlier reactive adverse events analyses. This section reviews such recent work on the phenomenon of breakdowns at large-scale – at micro-system interfaces in the surgical process, and notes the proposed recommendations for improvement, where applicable.

The work of Shultz et al. focused on pre-operative surgical work [254], specifically on the activities at the pre-admission unit. This work covers the patient preparation for surgery through several pathway steps up until the day before the actual surgical operation. Their study collected 49 hours of data on the sources of information, the facilitators and obstacles of information flow, and the known or likely consequences. They found that what facilitated information flow was recently performed test results, information from the patient's record/chart, and provider familiarity with specific patients. They also reported some problematic coordinations and information exchanges. For example, in the surgical unit of their study, information was often delayed or missing, unclear or incomplete, and not available when needed. Lack of communication was another disabler of information flow. The consequences were that decisions were delayed pending arrival of missing information and providers spent considerable time tracking down patient information. The authors recommended that the first step towards improving the perioperative process is to promote understanding of the upstream and downstream consequences of actions among surgical staff, as well as the benefits of team situational awareness.

The qualitative study of Christian, Roth and colleagues observed nine surgeries with an even more comprehensive approach. In their study, two observers collected field notes simultaneously at two separate locations: in the pre-operative area as patients were prepared for surgery, and in the OR while the room was being prepared for procedures [53, 246]. Their findings correspond to those of previous research – patient safety and case progression were compromised by two major factors: communication and information flow, and coordination of workload. Communication and information flow was particularly affected by issues related to handoffs in care, while coordination of workload by multiple competing tasks. One class of information loss identified was related to the dissemination of results of pre-operative assessments – for example, information from the surgeon's office, the consultant's office, or the pre-anesthesia testing unit was missing (*e.g.* consent documents). In other cases, the information was available but not attended to until very late into the patient preparation. Another class of information loss was the inadequate communication of the surgical plan to members of the OR team such that the nurses in the OR were uncertain of the details of the procedure to be performed and consequently of the preparation requirements. A third class of breakdowns resulted from the communications during patient handoff from the OR to the post-operative team. The cost of information loss was delays – from 0.5 to 4 hours, last minute changes in protocol, overuse of staff and resources, uncertainty in clinical decision making and planning, and oversight in patient preparation. The researchers concluded that candidate interventions for improvement of information flow were the surgery booking process, dissemination of surgery information, collaborative perioperative planning, and a standardized post-operative care reporting process.

Ren et al. examined coordination breakdowns in the work of multiple teams participating in the provision of surgical care in two hospitals [243]. Through 195 hours of observations and interviews, the researchers found that the majority of breakdowns occur at group boundaries. Coordination breakdowns were reported to occur anytime and anywhere in the surgical process. The sources of breakdowns were emergency cases, unexpected changes in patient condition, the absence of physicians and others due to unanticipated circumstances, lack of knowledge of organizational culture from novice staff, and inadequate staffing. As was the case in other studies, the consequences were delays, interpersonal tension, and conflict across groups. The authors envisioned the introduction of context-aware systems to improve inter-team coordination by promoting situation awareness throughout the surgical process.

A retrospective study conducted by Greenberg et al. reviewed 444 surgical malpractice claims and found a total of 60 cases in which communication breakdowns resulted in harm to the patient [108]. There were a total of 81 communication breakdowns, meaning that some cases experienced more than one communication failure. It was determined that breakdowns occurred throughout the surgical process – in the pre-operative (38%), operative (30%), and post-operative (32%) stages. The factors associated with breakdowns leading to patient injury were: status asymmetry between agents; ambiguity about roles, responsibilities, and leadership; handoff among providers; and transfer of the patient from one point of care to another. In order to prevent breakdowns, the authors advised the following: implementation of triggers to mandate communication, structured handoff and transfer protocols, and standard use of read-backs.

Some preliminary work is also worth mentioning. Healey et al. speculate that there may be as many as 149 failure modes in the transfer of information across the phases of elective surgery [127]. Other preliminary findings reported in [307] identify breakdowns in surgical care to be: blood not sent for testing, results not sent to the OR, add-on case did not have enough information, patient blood type is unknown, no blood available, and surgery continues longer than expected.

The studies reviewed in this section represent the few investigations currently available on macro-system level breakdowns in perioperative work. Being pioneers in this endeavor, these types of studies have yet to mature – the reported findings in the aforementioned ethnographic research (Greenberg's retrospective study excluded from this category) were based on observational notes and on interviews. Hence, no formal data coding and analysis were applied in this research. The reports were qualitative descriptions of observed phenomena. Only Shultz's study [254] ventured slightly beyond descriptions – the researchers categorized breakdowns at the inter-team level according to their criteria of interest and produced frequencies of observed types of breakdowns and their consequences. However, no mapping between breakdowns and consequences was provided.

This book is possibly the first to take a mixed methods design approach to the study of breakdowns at large in the surgical process. By doing so the strength of quantitative inquiry is used to provide meaningful insights as to the relationship between coordination mechanisms and breakdown properties, while the qualitative analysis complements these insights with the exploration of underlying reasons for the quantitative findings. Two theoretical models are derived to aid the understanding of breakdowns. The first conceptualizes the relationship between coordination mechanisms at work and breakdowns. The second implicates the association of breakdowns and safety. This book takes an even farther step in using the findings about breakdowns at large in perioperative work to deduct a breakdown detection method and a design framework.

Past work has shown that progress comes from going beyond surface descriptions to discover underlying patterns of systemic factors [303], *i.e.* genotypes – patterns of how people, teams, and organizations coordinate activities, information and problem solving to cope with the complexities of problems [138]. Research on patient safety should be using and expanding the set of genotypical patterns related to breakdowns that occur in health settings [303]. This book advances the current knowledge in this direction.

2.3.3 Breakdown detection

In order to improve safety, a better understanding of and support for breakdown management is needed. Achieving effective breakdown detection at the macro-system level is the first step towards this goal. As the field of patient safety has only recently emerged, research has yet to address this promising avenue towards improving safety. The goal of this book is, therefore, to contribute to the development of a breakdown management framework based on a review of breakdown detection approaches in domains that have already invested in research on detection. Following the review, this book proposes and validates a method for breakdown detection that is adjusted to the requirements of analysis of inter-team breakdowns in surgical care.

2.3.4 Approaches to the study of breakdowns in surgical care

Although breakdowns have been identified as the leading cause of adverse events, most studies of breakdowns reported in the literature are reactive in nature, i.e. post hoc event analyses [1, 145, 157, 226, 276]. The advantage of reactive retrospective analyses is the identification of specific factors that contribute to a particular type of breakdown. The disadvantage is that this type of analysis does not address latent conditions predisposing to types of breakdowns that have not occurred in the past. Further, the depth and scope of retrospective analysis has been questioned. Some have raised concerns about this type of analysis since its effectiveness is dependent on the information archived, the memory for past events and conditions, and the current understanding of tasks and human performance [125]. It is advised that many aspects of the system that may influence performance are not measurable retrospectively.

Very few studies (those reviewed earlier in this chapter) have taken on the proactive task of exploring breakdown conditions and processes in the surgical setting, as they occur in daily practice – i.e. as latent factors that did not necessarily manifest themselves as serious adverse events. These prospective studies looked at communication and coordination patterns, human errors, efficiencies and inefficiencies in team dynamics. They identified patterns of problematic communication and types of critical situations when breakdowns occur. With a retrospective approach, the majority of communication issues identified through the work reviewed earlier in this chapter would not be considered at all, as the breakdowns never materialized into adverse events. By examining prospectively the circumstances before, during and after a specific breakdown, a more precise recreation of the event can be described, including the contributing factors [53]. Another significant advantage of investigating in a prospective manner is that the influence of risk factors such as litigation, recrimination, feeling of guilt and shame are avoided [276]. As the social and organizational precursors to less severe events are similar or the same as those to adverse events, the unsafe features of organizations can be highlighted before a serious incident occurs.

Patient safety demands design of systems to make risky interventions reliable [86]. It has been argued that high reliability organizations take a proactive approach to breakdown management. This approach contrasts with the predominantly reactive approach in healthcare [142] that focuses on preventing the recurrence of adverse events [38]. Resilient organizations successfully detect dangerous conditions and adapt to absorb variations, changes and disruptions before serious harmful consequences arise [225]. Breakdown detection enables a-priori breakdown management measures, avoiding the negative effect of an accident such as patient harm, litigation, feelings of guilt, shame, etc.

Another consideration in the study of breakdowns is the scope of analysis. As discussed earlier, despite the adoption of a systems perspective, the majority of research so far has been focused on the operating theatre micro-system. Further, most of the measures and interventions developed have focused on the human agents rather than the processes and the information and communication needs. For example, the human-centered systems approach to the study of errors in hospitals has been fixed on the cognitive aspects of the human in her interaction with the external system – hence, the focus on slips, lapses and mistakes, as well as on skills, rules and knowledge. However, the causes of communication failure go beyond interactions and their relationship to human cognition, and derive from the design of the team processes and technology [127]. Thus, there is a call for expansion of the human-centered focus of analysis to become process-oriented as well. At a minimum, the focus of analysis should take into account the surgical care continuum, including technical and administrative aspects, communication culture, process structure, and coordination architecture.

Last but not least, the study of breakdowns will benefit from the complementary utilization of qualitative and quantitative investigative techniques. The review of the literature testifies to the fact that so far the problem has been addressed mostly qualitatively. To gain predictive and generalization power, research on breakdowns in surgical care must also include sound quantitative analyses.

This book integrates a prospective approach with a process-oriented perspective. Further, this book presents the analysis of breakdowns in two hospitals with the depth offered by qualitative methods and the power of statistical inference.

2.4 Breakdowns framework and hypotheses

Based on the existing body of knowledge on essential communication processes in surgical settings, as well as knowledge on active and latent contributors to breakdowns in perioperative processes, this section derives a basic set of properties of breakdowns and repairs (the measurement units for these properties are elaborated on in Chapter 3, Section 3.3.5). Six hypotheses are also inductively developed regarding the interrelationships between breakdown properties and their respective repairs.

2.4.1 Breakdown properties

Previous work showed that the tangible aspects of coordination, such as the utilization of physical objects or artifacts to support collaborative work, are at the core of managing coordination in clinical work in OR suites [305, 312]. In addition, object and artifact affordances had profound implications for both the efficiency of coordination and for the development of information and communication technology [305]. In a study of patient handoffs, Wilson et al. [301] found that changing the nature of the coordination tool from a paper summary sheet to a digital display - i.e. from a physical loosely private artifact to a public display – resulted in new access patterns to the information regarding patient handoffs. These new access patterns changed the purpose of the tool from one of coordination to one of reporting (an unintended design consequence). In other studies, clinicians were seen to print out the list of patients under their care, despite the fact that the list was available on their electronic application [272, 305,

312]. Cultural norms, the intangible coordinating conventions, were also shown to be prominent in all medical settings [59, 112]. These studies highlight the significance of the tangible and intangible aspects of clinical work. Therefore, based on these insights, we conclude that tangibility should be considered as one of the critical properties of coordination, and consequently of coordination breakdowns.

Proposition (A): The tangibility of the coordination mechanism employed is an important property of coordination breakdowns.

Field studies in various OR suites revealed a number of persistent categories of information that trigger coordination and communication efforts – e.g. information regarding the surgical schedule, staffing, room assignment, equipment, patient preparedness, and others [200, 201, 206, 243]. These categories are referred to as 'themes'. While the patterns of communication could vary based on the characteristics of the organizational process, the themes transcend particular settings [200]. Themes of coordination are identified through observable communication episodes. In turn, the frequency, timeliness, and accuracy of communication determines the quality and efficiency of patient care [105]. The above empirical studies suggest that if breakdowns in patient care should occur, the communication episodes related to these breakdowns would expose a particular theme related to each breakdown, from a set of common themes of surgical coordination. Thus, it is deduced that:

Proposition (B): A breakdown is characterized by a theme.

Investigations of adverse events in healthcare have usually found one of three types of root causes behind accidents – communication/coordination breakdowns, human/use errors, or technical/device failures [1, 145, 157, 276]. Hence, breakdowns can be typified according to their root cause.

Proposition (C): A breakdown is characterized by a type.

The scale of coordination – intra-team or inter-team (*i.e.* micro- or macro-system related) – in relation to breakdowns has not been explored as a variable in previous studies of surgical settings. As discussed earlier in this chapter, the majority of such studies focused on breakdowns in teamwork (*i.e.* intra-team), while only a few looked at potential issues at the inter-team level, but did not establish a relationship between these issues and other characteristics of perioperative work. However, studies in organization science have brought an appreciation of the differences in coordination at each scale level within work organizations [298]. Therefore, it is proposed that coordination scale be a property of breakdowns.

Proposition (D): A breakdown is characterized by its relevance to coordination scale.

This book also suggests that a breakdown can be described in terms of its lifetime – the distance traveled from origin of breakdown to detection, and to repair location in the process (The construct of distance is left open-ended here. A distance metric for this research is specified in Chapter 3, Section 3.3.5).

Proposition (E): A breakdown is characterized by a lifetime.

The property of breakdown theme could be seen as a refinement of breakdown type. Also coordination scale could roughly reflect the distance described by the breakdown lifetime. In this sense, these two dyads are not completely independent of each other. Therefore, an inherent relationship can be assumed between coordination scale and breakdown lifetime, as well as between type and theme. Thus, a statistical association for these dyads should not be sought in the study of breakdowns. The rest of the properties are fundamentally unique meta-descriptions of underlying mechanisms (e.g. information need, organizational level, tangible aspects) that are not related to each other and therefore statistical correlations among them are allowed. The allowable correlations between breakdown properties are shown in Table 1.

Table 1. Allowable correlations between breakdown properties. X= allowable.

	tangibility	coordination scale	breakdown lifetime	type	theme
tangibility		X	X	X	X
coordination scale	X			X	X
breakdown lifetime	X			X	X
type	X	X	X		
theme	X	X	X		

Based on the above assumptions, the following hypotheses are concluded:

Hypothesis 1: Tangibility of coordination processes relates to breakdown theme.
Hypothesis 2: Tangibility of coordination processes relates to coordination scale (inter, intra, or both).

2.4.2 Repair properties

Breakdowns reflect misalignment of information between components of a socio-technical system, i.e. loss of common ground [54]. Thus, breakdowns trigger repair work related to information re-alignment. Such repair work can be described as being either information push or information pull. The chosen strategy can have profound significance for the (re-)design of processes and information technology. Therefore, repair strategy is defined as a property of breakdown repairs.

Proposition (F): Repairs are characterized by a repair strategy.

Repairs, being an overhead to regular work activities, incur some *cost* to fix the associated breakdown [121] (the notion of cost is open-ended here - a particular cost metric is chosen in Chapter 3, Section 3.3.5). Hence, it is suggested that repair cost is an attribute of repairs.

Proposition (G): Repairs can be characterized by a repair cost.

Repairs are consequences of breakdowns. Thus, repairs are hypothesized to be derivatives of breakdown properties. Therefore, the following hypotheses are inferred:

Hypothesis 3: Tangibility of coordination mechanism relates to the type of repair strategy employed.
Hypothesis 4: Breakdown type relates to repair strategy.
Hypothesis 5: Breakdown theme relates to repair strategy.
Hypothesis 6: Breakdown lifetime (origin-detection-repair) correlates to repair cost.

2.5 The significance of technology design and processes

The role of technology in facilitating errors that result in patient complications and death has been a major concern for the past two decades. Design decisions that neglect existing work practices or knowledge on human cognition processes are the root causes of adverse events associated with technology use in the clinical setting. Computer displays, interfaces and devices in healthcare exhibit classic human-computer interaction deficiencies [303]. There is also a concern that the calls for increased use of integrated computerized information systems to reduce error introduces new and predictable forms of error unless there is a significant investment in user-centered design [303].

Hospitals are fragmented socio-technical systems [305], and technology is currently adopted at the departmental/unit level, instead of through the continuum of patient care. The situation triggers both technical and communication issues with impact on quality and safety of care, while de-contextualized metrics of adoption describe implementations as successful (This point is elaborated on in Section 2.5.2).

In some adverse events, direct active conditions related to interface design can be traced to have interplayed with human cognition at human-computer interaction time to cause fatal accidents – *e.g.* the administration of a lethal overdose of radiation [48]. These errors are known as use errors - a pattern of predictable human errors that can be attributed to inadequate or improper design [145]. In other cases, the reasons lie at the intersection of a web of latent conditions - poorly integrated technology and existing process, procedure, culture and other socio-technical factors. Thus, the idea that social-organizational theory must be considered in technology design and evaluation has recently gained prominence.

Barley conducted one of the very early studies on the effects of technology introduction into clinical work [30, 31]. Specifically, he examined the introduction of identical technology in two hospitals and found that the socio-organizational effects were considerably different. His ethnographic observations followed the time 'before, during and after' the first CT scanner machine was purchased in both hospitals. Barley reported the tremendous impact of introducing the technology on social order and work structure. The new technology affected skills and expertise required in clinical work, which consequently affected behavior patterns. In the first hospital the new technology challenged the hierarchical status quo and shifted the powers of autonomy from radiologists to technologists. This change created tensions that were later resolved by a further restructuring of the division of responsibilities. In the second hospital the new technology reinforced the culture of hierarchical division between radiologists and technologists, which resulted in a reduction of autonomy for the technologists. In both hospitals, traditional roles and patterns of interaction were altered through an evolution of work relationships.

A more recent study by Ash and colleagues examined the latent or silent errors that result from a mismatch between the functioning of patient care information systems and real-life demands of healthcare work [24]. Two main categories of latent errors that occur at the interface of the information system and clinical work practice were described: errors in the process of entering and retrieving information in or from the system, and errors in the communication and coordination processes that the system was supposed to support. In the latter case – of communication and coordination problems, there were two overarching issues: (1) misrepresenting collective, interactive work as a linear, clear-cut, and predictable workflow; and (2) misrepresenting communication as information transfer. Such failures are the result of mistaken assumptions about healthcare work that are built into patient care information systems, creating dysfunctional interactions with users and, sometimes, leading to actual errors in the provision of patient care.

Another study by Koppel et al. of hospital staff interaction with a widely used computerized provider order entry (CPOE) system found that the technology facilitated 22 types of medication error risks [160] – *e.g.* computer interaction procedures that do not correspond to work organization or usual behaviors, wrong patient or medication selection, inflexible ordering screens generating wrong orders, fragmented CPOE displays that prevent a coherent view of patients' medications, pharmacy inventory displays mistaken for dosage guidelines and others. Three quarters of the hospital staff reported observing each of these error risks, indicating that they occur weekly or more often.

In a recent survey of 176 U.S. hospitals that have implemented CPOE systems, it was reported that significant and widespread unintended negative consequences surfaced as a result of the technology implementation [26]. Over 73% of hospital respondents said that more work was created – *e.g.* the interface called for more steps in ordering for non-standard cases, some tasks became more difficult, the computer forced the user to complete all steps, etc. Further, 87% of hospitals experienced a significant workflow change, which resulted in some improvements. However, there were also negative effects, especially in the workflow of physicians who were forced to spend longer time ordering. Half of the hospitals also reported that the CPOE system resulted in inadequate communication between providers that necessitated the initiation of efforts at educating clinicians not to rely solely on the system. New patient safety issues were introduced as well, such as orders on the wrong patient, overlapping medication orders, desensitization to alerts, etc.

A qualitative research study by Edmondson and colleagues on introduction of minimally invasive technology into the cardiac OR in 16 hospitals reported significant effects on teamwork behaviors across organizations – tasks were changed, roles were blurred, task interdependency and consequently coordination demand were increased [82, 83]. In addition, there was a change in the power dynamic between the surgeon and the team – the surgeon's role shifted from one of an order giver to a team member. Overall, the difficulty encountered by clinicians was more behavioral than technical. Existing routines and status relationships presented powerful barriers to adoption. The researchers identified the crucial conditions for successful adoption of the new technology to be related to the management of the change and learning process, the quality of teamwork, and the leadership skills of the team leader in the OR (the surgeon).

Finally, despite the worldwide push towards digitizing medical records, including a recently passed healthcare legislation and stimulus package in the U.S., progress towards shared electronic health records has so far fallen short of expectations [85]. In addition, studies cast doubt whether it is possible to build information communication systems that actually improve integrated care [119, 122].

The significance of technology design in the provision of safety, quality and efficiency in patient care is critical. Improving design and implementation processes for clinical technology has been a major concern in recent years for both industry and research. A growing recognition of the complexity of the clinical setting and work has prompted an appreciation of social, organizational, professional, and other contextual considerations in design [140, 152, 242]. It has been advised that systems should be designed to support communication and provide the flexibility that is needed for them to better fit real work practices [24]. Further, it has been recommended that for automation concerned with information processing and decision making to be successful, the key requirement is to design for fluent, coordinated interaction between the human and machine elements of the system [303]. Although clinical care technology is rapidly improving, known design principles are still not evident in today's systems [24], which has resulted in slow adoption. To address some of the challenges, recently the AHRQ recommended that usability become part of the electronic patient record certification process [19].

2.5.1 The design process

The development activities in clinical technology design are fundamentally the same as in other domains [204]. Since comprehensive clinical domain standards are lacking, design practice relies on generic methods from the fields of Human Computer Interaction (HCI) and Computer Supported Cooperative Work (CSCW) [19, 149, 204, 228, 251, 253]. These methods are employed to derive user and interaction models, and produce concept designs. The typical waterfall model of sequential activities in the product development lifecycle is widely employed. Projects start with the conceptual phase, which is followed by data gathering to understand user needs. Task analyses, user profiling and occasionally field studies are conducted. Often, however, domain experts are utilized in place of actual users due to intellectual property and corporate privacy concerns. User needs are documented in high-level technical descriptions. Next, detailed requirements are generated. The design stage starts and early prototypes are then produced that get iterated as the project progresses to beta versions that ultimately lead to the final released product. Initial usability evaluation is performed with human factors experts or with users interacting with high fidelity prototypes. After the development of the complete system, further usability testing may be employed and regulatory technology certification is obtained. Figure 3 illustrates the process.

There are several differences from the typical development cycle. For example, regulatory approval needs to be obtained before a system is released. This step necessitates the incorporation of risk analysis, evaluation, and mitigation design activities. In addition, post-market field studies are conducted to understand product acceptance and safety in more detail [212].

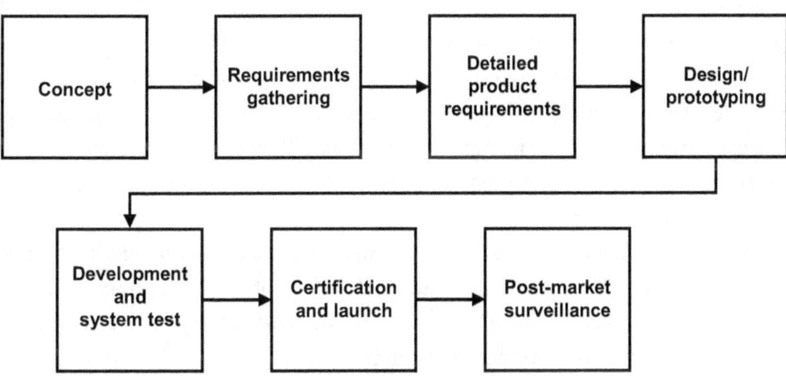

Figure 3: Product development lifecycle for clinical systems (Adapted from [204]).

Risk analysis is the investigation of available information to identify hazards and estimate risk [204]. It can include the use of tools such as Fault Tree Analysis or Failure Mode and Effects Analysis (see Appendix D.1). The estimation of risk may be qualitative and/or quantitative. The focus is on user error [145]. The analysis is conducted by performing an anticipative analysis of potential human errors for each of the tasks in the task analysis and by estimation of the frequency of occurrence of the errors and their severity. Once these factors are considered, a risk index is calculated.

Because of the safety risks posed, the FDA and other international bodies – IEC, ISO, AAMI, etc. have made human factors and usability engineering processes a priority for medical manufacturers [204]. In addition, these institutions have issued guidances and standards prescribing design activities (e.g. [2, 5, 8, 16, 18]). These are human factors design process guidelines for medical devices that advise on the consideration of cognitive and environmental factors that can influence human performance during interaction with a computer system. A good human factors engineering analysis for medical devices or software systems includes four major components: user, functional, task and representational analyses [318].

In terms of evaluation and mitigation design activities, usability evaluation has become an important validation tool [19]. There are two major approaches to evaluation – heuristic techniques and user testing. Heuristic evaluation techniques have gained prominence as an easy to use, easy to learn, discount and informal usability evaluation method [318]. Heuristic evaluation involves a representational user and a real computer. A small set of human factors experts examine the interface and judge its compliance with recognized usability principles, *i.e.* the heuristics [100]. A typical set of heuristics is the ten principles proposed by Nielsen and Molich [211]: simple and natural dialog, speaks the user's language, minimizes user memory load, is consistent, provide feedback, provide clearly marked exits, provide shortcuts, provide good error messages, prevent errors, provide help and documentation. Zhang et al. have modified and extended the common heuristics from usability engineering for use in the healthcare sector [318].

User testing involves a real system and real users interacting with a real computer [100]. The testing is conducted in a usability laboratory, where the methods of user performance measurement, think-aloud protocol collection and scenario-based usability testing can be used.

Heuristic evaluation and user testing are complementary as they are effective at identifying distinct sets of problems [100, 318]. The former predicts usability problems that more advanced users will experience. The latter identifies problems that novice users will encounter.

Methodological considerations and challenges

Although medical use errors (*i.e.* design-induced errors) have been a pressing issue for two decades [40, 41, 157], there still is no framework for design tailored to the requirements of the clinical domain. Current practice of design for medical applications relies on generic methodologies from the fields of HCI and groupware design [19, 149, 204, 228, 251, 253, 303]. Generic methods, however, are based on the assumption of an idealized workflow process – i.e. an ideal or expert user and a perfect progression along a formalized multi-path workflow specification. This contrasts with the expected reality at the end-user clinical domain. As was described earlier, the clinical setting, specifically surgical work, is characterized by a great deal of uncertainty. Another shortcoming of generic

HCI methods is that they are inadequate in expressing the complexity of clinical work [84]. Recent research on safety and quality in healthcare identified a number of factors that influence clinical practice – patient factors, task factors (*i.e.* use of protocols), individual factors (*e.g.* skills, competence, etc.), team factors, work environment, and institutional environment [232, 287]. It is suggested that relying on one level of improvement intervention while neglecting other important factors that influence clinical work will result in limited impact [287].

Generic groupware task-based design modeling methods and error analysis techniques currently applied in medical design are inadequate to meet the requirements of the domain. Methods such as Concur Task Tree (CTT) [223], Coordination, Cooperation und Communication (K3) [156], Groupware task analysis (GTA) [282], and Multiple Aspect Based Task Analysis (MABTA) [175] focus on taskwork, emphasize the importance of cooperation and contextual factors from the viewpoint of individual human actors, but fail to consider actual collaborative group processes [271] (i.e. a more global view of the system) or the role of technology in performing the activity. As a result of this overall situation, system development in healthcare is primarily focused on the individual healthcare professional [253]. The Collaborative Usability Analysis technique is the only one that shifts the focus of analysis from taskwork to teamwork [229]. All of the methods provide systematic formal models, but they do not account for the social processes that have significant safety implications. Further, present task modeling techniques offer limited expressiveness and medical application designers struggle to reflect numerous system components with their respective states and user tools within the task representations. Given the cooperative nature of contemporary healthcare and the significant role of technology in it, there is a need for an integrated approach of analysis that incorporates cooperative processes, safety, usability, and technology. This type of approach requires a level of analysis that synthesizes the individual, group, and organizational levels.

In healthcare, as in other domains, consideration of human factors comes during the late stages of IT-system evaluation and standardization compliance, but coordination breakdowns are beyond the scope of analyses. While there is an awareness of and emphasis on addressing user issues, the problems are still addressed at the final development stages – an approach that has proven expensive and ineffective in the software industry (see Appendix D.1). Human error is approached in an informal non-systematic way, preference testing is often applied [146], and human factors are considered at the representational level – through the lens of heuristic evaluations [318], and other usability criteria without respect to risk [146]. To make matters worse, heuristic evaluation deals only with a fraction of usability issues and is characterized by low validity [55, 100, 318].

Lab user testing is employed during final stages of system evaluation when major changes to design are beyond scope [204]. During the late stages of development, the issue of safety is addressed by means of standardization compliance and by post-market surveillance [204, 212]. This practice has proven inadequate for the production of safe and usable medical systems for high-risk environments.

Coordination requirements are not exploited in design of clinical systems nor are they conceptualized in design, and relevant breakdowns (especially related to inter-team macro-system level processes) are difficult to predict during risk analysis and to trigger in the course of user testing. There are also no design standards to guide the evaluation of technology designs and their impact on coordination processes. Requirements elicitation is still often performed according to conventional system development processes, reducing user involvement to user questionnaires and the like, rather than effectively analyzing the user needs in the context of social and organizational issues [253]. Moreover, the fact that technology integration will change work practices is often neglected.

A further problem in design practice for clinical systems is the utilization of domain experts in place of actual users due to intellectual property and corporate privacy concerns. Vendors assume that deriving user needs and requirements through the lens of domain experts will translate into the system integrating well in the field. However, the way people are supposed to work in theory never matches reality. Hence, the more specialized the system, the more user research is needed to ensure success [210]. If real users are not testing the system, there is a high probability that a plethora of usability problems will surface.

The concern for intellectual property and corporate privacy also determines the utilization of the waterfall model of development This is true despite the fact that this approach is not optimal since it creates the opportunity for incorrect design due to minimal user involvement. In the software industry, the iterative and participatory models of development are now widely used. These models include user involvement throughout the development lifecycle.

Some initial efforts to develop methods and techniques customized to meet the demands of design for clinical work have been made. For example, Zhang et al. modified Nielsen's usability heuristics to address human factors issues at the representational level of medical interface design [318]. However, as noted earlier, heuristic evaluation deals with a fraction of usability issues and is characterized by low validity [55, 100, 318]. Further, heuristic evaluation focuses on a single device or application and may not identify problems that arise because of the device's use environment [318]. Several other authors have drawn on their findings to derive functional requirements for technology. For instance, Seagull and colleagues recommended that to support schedule coordination in an OR environment, any new technology system must serve as a common referent for communication, provide a communal memory tool for planning, serve as catalyst for collaborative and distributed cognition, allow parallel manipulation for multiple user-groups, and allow flexible content reconfiguration [255]. Xiao noted that the tangible nature of healthcare delivery creates a challenge in bridging the gap between the tangible and virtual [305]. He proposed that to harness the potential of technology in supporting work in healthcare, the focus should be directed to the tangible aspects of work in modeling, designing, and supporting workflow. Specifically, the development of user requirements should take into account how artifacts are used and exploited to facilitate collaboration. Then, the design and deployment of new technology should support the functions provided by physical artifacts replaced or disrupted by new technology.

Though these recommendations address some methodological concerns, there is no design method in the literature that is specifically tailored to development work for the perioperative setting and is informed by the research in the domain. This book begins by using previous research to further the understanding of coordination in surgical work. Then, based on the existing and newly acquired knowledge, the book extrapolates system design guidelines and integrates them into a framework for design specific to surgical systems.

2.5.2 Adoption of electronic shared displays for coordination of patient care

Technology implementation in healthcare clinical environments is a challenging issue from a design and safety perspective. In recent years, the literature has abounded with examples of partially successful implementations that result in resistance to adoption, increased patient safety concerns, and changed workflows in unanticipated ways [160, 319]. The introduction of technology into the healthcare clinical environment has been shown to change clinical patient care in ways that prevent communication of important psycho-social patient parameters [319], to create conditions predisposing to medical errors [160], to desensitize clinicians to alerts [275], or to change the nature of collaborative work such as the task of handover [301]. The most common and overt consequences of technology introduction include: incurred investment overhead of increased demand for training, repeated rollouts, costly training, as well as workarounds devised by end-users that undermine the benefits of the implemented technology. Most importantly, technology implementations in healthcare are associated with poor patient outcomes (*e.g.* health complications and sometimes fatalities).

This book reports a longitudinal study that investigated the effects of the introduction of a communication technology – an electronic whiteboard (eWhiteboard) – into the surgical work process. Whiteboards are one of the most common and exploited communication tools in clinical work environments. In their analog form – i.e. erase boards, they have been shown to facilitate negotiation of scheduling, joint planning, inter-personal communication, and inter-group coordination in the clinical setting [103, 290, 308, 311]. Whiteboard's large sizes enable instant and distal views from different locations and by multiple people [311]. A recent study showed that clinicians in an emergency department communicated in front of the whiteboard 24% of the time [89]. The importance of shared access to information in collaborative work, as well as the need for accurate and timely communication between care providers in healthcare have brought about the age of a welcome introduction of a new generation of whiteboards – the electronic ones. The advantages of such distributed shared access public displays in healthcare operations include synchronous communication, improved and standardized communication, improved group decision making, increased efficiency, and greater staff satisfaction [230, 302]. Often there is an assumption that the large interactional space afforded by a display only benefits the work practice [301]. However, there are serious concerns about privacy of patient information - whiteboards publicly display identifying patient information that a passing hospital visitor can see. On the other hand, if patient information is secured through the use of numeric patient identification or an alias, the usability and effectiveness of the system is reduced. This, in turn, can affect patient safety. Further, ethnographic studies in dynamic clinical environments continuously reveal that by changing the nature of communication from private to public, the new eWhiteboards transform the use of critical psycho-social information in clinical work in unanticipated ways [301, 319]. For instance, Wilson et al.'s study of the effects of introduction of a large shared display into the pediatric unit found that the public display resulted in greater scrutiny of the patient information and patient care work documented for handover [301]. Consequently, the summary sheet was no longer a tool supporting the work of handover and the ongoing work of the shift, but a mechanism for submitting the work of the shift to the scrutiny of senior staff. The authors voiced their concern that the public display of the summary sheet might become an idealized record of the work rather than remain a useful and less formal artifact of work coordination. In summary, eWhiteboards fight design issues related to contextual use and care continuum implementation challenges much like other forms of clinical technology (*e.g.* medication administration and patient records systems).

One barrier to improving implemented patient coordination systems is that validated measures of adoption, satisfaction and efficiency seem to produce favorable outcomes. The availability of electronic data facilitates fast automated statistical reporting of business and quality metrics. The success of technology adoption in hospitals is often evaluated through the lens of such operational metrics - patient throughput, patient visit duration, clinical outcomes, and self-report evaluations. More often than not, these measures result in highly positive ratings. Additionally, such metrics confine analysis to the department/unit that integrated the new technology thereby neglecting problems at the continuum of care level. As a consequence, shortcomings of technologies are often overlooked and implementations are deemed successful.

It is only the field studies that identify issues with integration. The differing outcomes are due to the diverse nature of the measured parameters – metrics being concerned with de-contextualized aggregate data (*i.e.* automated reports) or reasoned/perceived use (*i.e.* surveys) vs. actual use [155]. Automated electronic data analysis lacks analytical and methodological concerns. In addition, survey techniques depend on subjective judgments that remain implicit in the data [80]. Field studies, on the other hand, reflect actual use in-context but generally are not part of current implementation processes, nor do they present convincing quantifiable data. Usability experts have noted, however, that valid data comes from what people do, not what they say [210].

The study by Munkvold et al. [203] illustrates the aforementioned concern very well. The research examined the introduction of an electronic patient record for coordination of handover in the Rheumatology department of a hospital. The project was proclaimed successful by an internal hospital evaluation based on nurses' self-reported work time activities and a questionnaire they filled out. The hospital's report stated reduction in time spent on handover and overtime reduction. The nurses were also more attentive to the written documentation and had become more structured in the way they documented their work – thus the quality of the documentation was improved. Statistical figures and the nurses confirmed that the objectives were reached. However, the observations of actual work conducted by the researchers revealed a different reality – formalizing the nursing handover through the introduction of the system with the goal to reduce redundancy had in fact resulted in re-allocation of the redundancy to a different time in the work, into different artifacts, and onto old artifacts that were now utilized differently. For example, the introduction of the electronic system resulted in fragmentation of the patient 'story' among different people and artifacts. In turn, this development necessitated the introduction of a weekly summary record integrating information on patients in the ward.

In this book, a longitudinal study of surgical patient care coordination examines the coordination breakdowns prior to and post eWhiteboard implementation. The study is unique in that it focuses specifically on the evolution of breakdowns through the technology integration, rather than studying its effects in an exploratory manner as previous research has done. In this book, adoption/satisfaction self-reports and observational findings are juxtaposed by quantifying actual eWhiteboard use. The study explores the complex interplay between improved patient care communication through the eWhiteboard, increased breakdowns occurrence, and reports of high satisfaction with the technology. The research finds that the lack of trust among teams of clinical care is a major disabler of adoption of the eWhiteboard.

2.6 Conclusion

In order to address potential safety, quality, and efficiency issues inherent in proximal and latent healthcare system factors, there is a need for improved understanding of breakdowns in healthcare processes through systematic formal studies that go beyond qualitative descriptions of observed phenomena and address breakdowns at the system level [38, 45]. Further, operational efficiency in hospitals will be enhanced by a recognition of the factors that contribute to breakdowns and by eliminating costly repair overhead. [181]. The fundamental value of an appreciation of the deep features of breakdowns and respective repairs is that it is a rich resource for human- and process-centered information technology system design solutions [29, 99, 217]. Thus, the goal of this book is to acquire knowledge about breakdowns and to use it to inform and improve the design methods for surgical care systems. By addressing breakdowns in clinical work during the early stages of system design, future technology will adequately meet the communication and coordination demands of clinical work. As a result, adoption and safety will be enhanced.

3

Process-oriented empirical study

This chapter provides a detailed overview of the research methodology. First, the choice of research design is justified and the theoretical framework explained. Next, the two hospitals' profiles are presented. The chapter then continues with a detailed description of the data collection procedures and tools, the coding scheme, the resulting data sets, and the analysis methods.

To address the research problems of this book, it was necessary to examine breakdowns in more than one hospital and to study the evolution of breakdowns through the lens of technology integration in a longitudinal fashion. Below, three studies that make up this work are presented. Two of the studies took place in the same hospital, the third in a different hospital. The data collection in the first hospital proceeded in two phases – before the introduction of an electronic whiteboard communication tool (Phase 1) and eight months after its integration into the perioperative work process (Phase 2). Only one study in the second hospital was conducted. In all studies the data collection approach was identical - nurses, personal assistants, coordinators, physicians, administrators, etc. were observed as they performed their routine work throughout the surgical journey areas providing care for patients who have surgery.

The majority of the results, presented in the next chapter, are concerned with the comparison of breakdowns in the two hospitals. To that end, the two data sets from the first hospital are integrated to produce a unified picture of the state of breakdowns in that hospital. The results are derived from statistical analysis of the coded breakdowns data (the coding scheme is explained in this chapter and the coded data can be found in Appendix B.2). For the purpose of discussion of the technology adoption study, the two datasets are considered individually and juxtaposed.

3.1 Research methodology design

Choosing a research methodology appropriate to the research question, and informed by a theoretical foundation, is critical [43]. To date, the research on patient safety has predominantly followed the qualitative research framework, utilizing the power of the narrative, the case studies - stories of adverse events to yield insights, provide pattern recognition for patient safety practitioners, and create a new cycle of improved understanding and system design [86]. Health technology assessment research also relies on qualitative methodologies [191]. While the qualitative approach provides rich understanding of a particular instance of a patient safety concern, it lacks generalizability and does not present quantifiable data often sought after in scientific disciplines. Some of the more recent research aiming to address this issue adopts a quantitative framework through survey methodologies that examine a problem across a great number of settings and organizations. This approach, however, cannot account for the complexity of underlying proximal and latent systems factors contributing to patient safety threats. Moreover, survey techniques depend on subjective judgments, which remain implicit in the data [80].

The research presented in this book adopts a mixed methods research design to the study of latent factors in patient safety – specifically to the problem of communication and coordination breakdowns across two settings, offering a richer description [22, 215], capturing a level of systems complexity reflective of the research question and environment under investigation. The goal in selecting a mixed methods research design was to acquire an in-depth understanding through comprehensive analysis, as well as a degree of generalizability of outcomes demonstrated through quantifiable data [67]. The integration of qualitative and quantitative techniques is not new in organizational and health services research [22, 90, 214]. The methodologies are considered complementary [187] because each compensates the other for its weaknesses. The integration of both approaches is performed during the interpretation of results [67].

This research utilized several tools in the conduct of the empirical study of communication and coordination breakdowns. First, a grounded theory exploratory approach was adopted [266] in the discovery of broad themes of coordination and information related to the occurrence of breakdowns in the surgical work practice, during observations. In previous studies (reviewed in Chapter 2), the grounded theory approach has been found useful. Also, prior-research-driven top-down thematic analysis [42, 43] facilitated the initial development of data codes (presented later in this chapter). In addition, a bottom-up thematic analysis [42, 43], also known as open coding [266], was followed for the development of further themes in the coding scheme via an inductive data-driven approach applied post-data collection. Finally, appropriate statistical analyses methods were utilized for the quantitative analysis of the coded data, as well as for the analysis of a survey. Figure 4 shows the methodology for the research in this book in the context of the thematic analysis process [43].

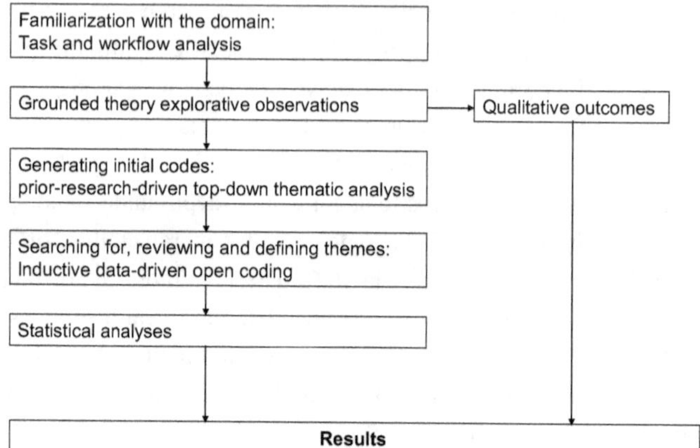

Figure 4: Research methodology.

3.1.1 Theoretical perspective

Through the lens of the Swiss cheese perspective (introduced in Chapter 2, Section 2.1.2), this book centers on the study of latent communication and coordination factors that have potential to affect patient safety downstream in the surgical process. The Swiss Cheese model was not applied in the analysis of breakdowns since its core concept requires that an event under consideration has transpired into an accident. Given that the scope of this study is the prospective investigation of latent factors, the model is not applicable. Nevertheless, it helps to understand the nature of the problem studied.

The theoretical assumptions that underpin the study design and analyses in this work come from the frameworks of activity theory, workflow analysis and systems engineering. Activity theory [153, 164] examines activity level behavior in relation to social factors such as the organization of labor, conflicts of interest, culture, etc. Activity theory's focus of analysis includes a cultural-historical perspective [60, 87] as rendered through the study of workers, task, and community. Interactions between a worker and a task are mediated by artifacts. Interactions between a worker and her community are mediated by procedures. Examining the use of artifacts and procedures in-situ allows researchers to extrapolate the effects of socio-technical system mechanisms on the entire socially distributed activity system [28]. Workflow analysis [34, 188, 194, 281], on the other hand, seeks an understanding of work products – material and conceptual, through the analysis of their transformations. The focus is centered on processes that influence the work, inputs/outputs to each step in a process, and on the impact and roles of people as they interact with the work products.

This book integrates the concepts of activity theory and workflow analysis in the study design and analyses. Observations and relevant data collection focus on conflicts of interest, examine the use of artifacts and coordinating procedures in-situ, and investigate the inputs and outputs of each process step. Further, the systems engineering framework directed the definition of the study design and analyses. The surgical micro-systems were modeled and analyzed. In addition, the coordination, synchronization and integration of the micro-systems were investigated in relation to breakdowns.

Overall, the ideas in this book are influenced by a multidisciplinary perspective stemming from the social and engineering disciplines. This perspective matches the relevant patient safety, human-computer interaction/usability, and systems engineering frameworks of research.

3.2 Research setting

The research was conducted within the busy elective surgery units of two urban teaching Canadian hospitals. The main criterion for selecting the hospitals was that the two organizations should be sufficiently different from one another in terms of their organizational culture, history, function and size. This condition was chosen for two reasons: 1) so that potential similarities between the organizations would have greater generalizability, and 2) so that potential differences can be explored in relation to breakdowns. The first hospital selected is a typical urban general medium-size institution with a specialization in neurology. It also belongs to a network of three university teaching hospitals. The second hospital chosen is a much larger institution with a religious affiliation (Catholic) that has historically determined the mission and provision of patient care services with an emphasis on compassion. This hospital specializes in trauma treatment for the city. Based on the above factors, it was deemed that a fundamental difference, culturally and functionally, exists between the two organizations. For privacy reasons, this book will refer to the hospitals as Hospital_1 and Hospital_2.

3.2.1 Hospital_1

Hospital_1, a 236 bed institution, offers a history of over a hundred years of urban patient care. Hospital_1 is a teaching hospital for a major university. Since the 1990s, the hospital has become the designated neurology center of excellence with the largest cluster of neuro-surgeons in the province. The elective surgery unit is comprised of 15 operating rooms and performs 50-80 surgeries per day, including emergency operations. The surgical division employs a total of 350 people – administrative and professional staff.

The surgical patient care flow for Hospital_1 is shown in Figure 5. Each box represents a micro-system, referred to as *point of care*, and represents a process carried out by a number of agents comprising a team and using artifacts and technologies. As can be seen in the figure, multiple teams (*i.e.* micro-systems) work synchronously and asynchronously to provide patient care. Each team is in a separate physical space. Therefore, depending on the focus of analysis, the coordination space properties can change from intra- to inter-team (or micro- to macro-system level). The OR Desk is served by a clerk who is the main coordinator of the process, and is the only agent who never treats patients. The clerk tracks and distributes the most up-to-date information on the state of affairs to all parties involved.

For the study, the majority of clinical and administrative staff working in the micro-systems under consideration volunteered to participate. The participant sample included 13 employees (out of a total of 15 in these micro-systems), both men and women.

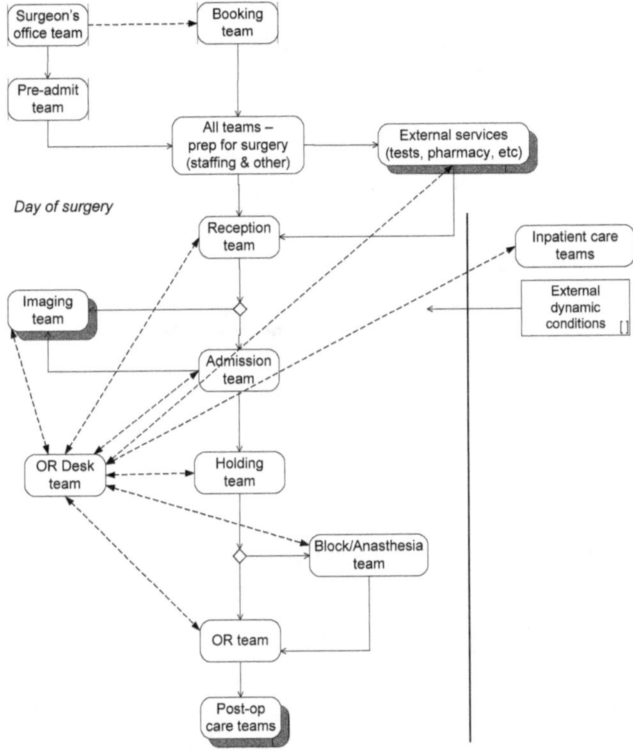

Figure 5: The observed surgical process workflow at Hospital_1. Shaded boxes represent optional workflow steps, and dotted lines indicate direct information/communication flow lines.

3.2.2 Hospital_2

Hospital_2, over one hundred years old, is a Catholic, teaching institution affiliated with a major university. Hosptial_2 is a busier healthcare provider with 900 beds. It is the designated adult trauma centre for the city. Hospital_2 runs 22 operating rooms and performs 55-90 surgeries per day, including emergency and trauma cases. Over 400 administrative and professional employees provide the perioperative services at the hospital.

Hospital_2's flow of patient care is very similar to that of Hospital_1, with the exception of the communication links. The flow is illustrated in Figure 6. Similar to Hospital_1, each point of care represented on the diagram is a micro-system – a process carried out by collaborating agents in a team. Artifacts and technologies mediate some of the work interactions and information exchanges. Teams are distributed in the physical space of the hospital. The OR desk at Hospital_2 is served by multiple clerks and a charge nurse - they coordinate the process by tracking information and negotiating decisions, and they do not treat patients.

Similar to Hospital_1, most nursing and administrative staff in the micro-systems under consideration volunteered to participate. The sample size was 18 employees (out of a total of 20 in these micro-systems), both men and women.

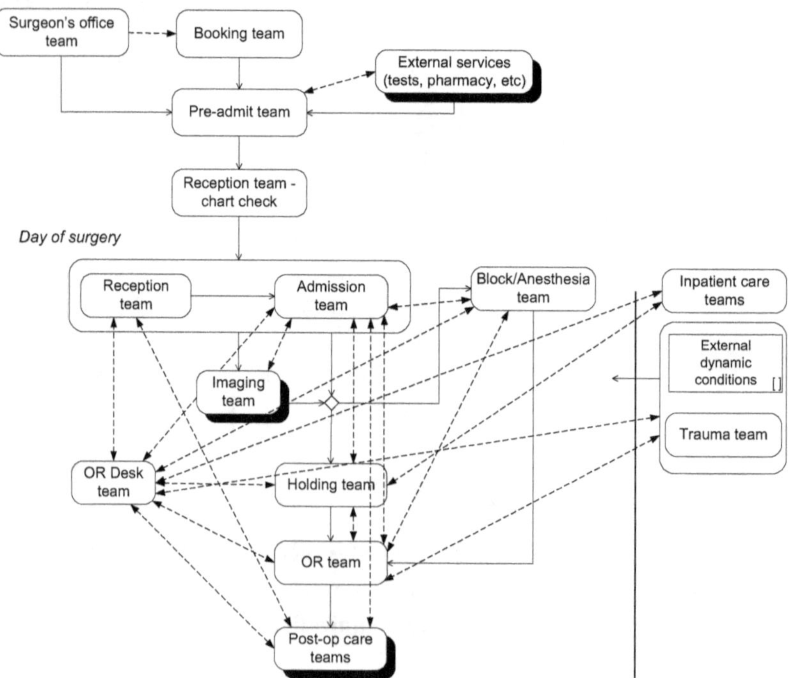

Figure 6: The observed surgical process workflow at Hospital_2. Shaded boxes represent optional workflow steps, and dotted lines indicate direct information/communication flow lines.

3.2.3 Process structure and communication flows

One notable difference between the patient care flow diagrams of the two hospitals studied is the established communication channels for information exchange and coordination among micro-systems. In Hospital_1, communication is centralized through the functional allocation of process coordination responsibility into the role of the OR desk clerk (Figure 5). Under normal circumstances, teams do not communicate directly. Each team contacts the OR desk clerk with questions or to pass important patient care information along to another team. The clerk is responsible for the distribution of information regarding changes in patient care to all parties involved. Communication in Hospital_1 is therefore formalized. The process structure provides streamlined communication that avoids variation in practice.

In Hospital_2, communication channels are less formalized. Direct communication channels among all teams exist (Figure 6). The OR desk team's responsibility for coordination of the process is limited to a few scenarios - for trauma and inpatient care coordination. For all other matters, teams communicate to each other directly as needed. Further, clinical staff from one team often help out with the work of another team through negotiated rotation hours during the day. Thus, the established process in Hospital_2 was designed to allow for greater flexibility and a lower level of formalism.

Another important communication flow difference between the two hospitals is in their communication culture – in Hospital_1 information is pushed through the system in a pre-emptive and proactive manner, while in Hospital_2 information is pulled when needed (*i.e.* in a reactive fashion).

3.3 Procedure and observational data collection

Ethics approval for the conduct of this work was obtained from each hospital (file #07-0719-AE for Hospital_1, and file #09-013 for Hospital_2) prior to the onset of the studies. Informational sessions were organized to introduce clinical and administrative staff to the study, its goals, methodologies and implications of participation. Participation was voluntary and almost all front-line staff in both surgical units enrolled. The participants included nurses, clinical and clerical staff at the elective surgery units whose functional roles were part of direct or indirect patient care, coordination and administration of the perioperative process.

3.3.1 Understanding the domain

The observations were conducted with a systems approach - they spanned the surgical process from surgery booking to patient reception at the OR: surgery booking, pre-admission consults, patient reception, admission, holding area, OR desk, and block/anesthesia room. First, the tasks and workflow of all agents in the surgical process were analyzed through a set of unstructured interviews and observations (a total of 21 hours in each hospital). In addition, diagrammatic descriptions of all functional roles in the surgical process activity were produced. Examples of the workflow models can be found in Appendix A.1 and of the task models in Appendix A.2. An advanced practice nurse with extensive surgical experience verified the correctness of the representations. This analysis facilitated a thorough understanding of the work practice and revealed that the majority of breakdowns do not become visible (i.e. are not detected) until the actual day of surgery, although they may have originated prior to that. Therefore, the consequent data collection efforts focused on the micro-systems relevant to the day the patient arrives for surgery, *i.e.* on the operative stage of the process. Further, understanding the work in each point of care facilitated the development of categories for quantitative data collection.

3.3.2 Data collection

As mentioned above, data collection efforts focused on the operative stage – the micro-systems relevant to the day when the patients arrive for surgery: patient reception, admission, holding area, OR desk, and block/anesthesia room. This included the time of anesthetizing the patient in the Block Room before the actual surgery. Clinicians were observed as they performed their routine work throughout the surgical journey areas. Observations took place in one micro-system, or point of care, at a time. About four full days of data collection were appropriated for each point of care in each study (data collection procedures are elaborated below). Clinical and administrative staff preparation activities for surgeries scheduled for the following day were also shadowed. Additionally, in Hospital_1, nine patients were followed from the moment of arrival in the hospital through their journey to the OR.

Observations started at 6am when the first patients arrive at the hospital and continued throughout the working day. Both high and low workload periods were observed in all patient care areas. The data collection spanned over three weeks for each of the three studies.

Numerous challenges exist in collecting a complete transcript of real-time events in the highly-intensive and dynamic surgical environment – chief amongst them are the legal and ethical obstacles in recording video and the incompleteness of observational notes. To circumvent these, a data collection platform was utilized in this research - the RATE tool [113]. RATE allows one to pre-program a number of communication and coordination related categories of interest. The tool enabled the collection of a complete time-stamped record of all interactions among clinicians and with physical and digital artifacts, at a low transcription cost of several mouse-clicks per event. The observer carried a laptop and recorded all interactions, including data on information flow and mediating artifacts. In-situ informal interviews with clinicians were performed to clarify actions, processes, intentions, and motivations.

3.3.3 Data collection coding scheme

A basic coding scheme for in-vivo data coding was developed with the goal to collect all communication events observed in a systematic fashion that will allow for qualitative and quantitative analysis. Each data entry included information on origin and target of communication, start and end time, event type, theme of coordination and medium. The main categories of data collection were the following:

Origin: the functional role initiating the communication

Target: the functional role receiving the communication

Event type: the type of communication event (e.g. update, planning, questioning)

Content: the theme of coordination; the specific reason for initiating this event (e.g. patient location, OR readiness, schedule)

Comments: a free field for any additional information; mostly used to indicate the specific medium or tool or artifact utilized

The RATE tool automatically time-stamped each recorded event. The events were encoded as database tuples where each category represented a field (*i.e.* attribute) that takes on a predefined set of nominal values. The values for each field can be found in Appendix A.3. The resulting observational data entries appeared in this form:

Start	End	Origin	Target	Event type	Content	Comments	Flag
11:30:07	11:30:14	Nurse5	None	outgoing call	OR readiness	phone	
11:30:18	11:30:40	OR desk	Nurse4	incoming call	patient status	phone	
11:30:30	11:30:39	None	Nurse4	artifact	None	chart	
11:30:42							breakdown

Breakdowns were flagged at start and end time. All events in-between were transcribed in detail and complemented with observer annotations where necessary. An open commenting field allowed the observer to also record unstructured information for additional thoroughness and clarity of the collected data. Breakdowns were further analyzed post data collection to determine the breakdown triggers, type of repair strategy employed, coordination mechanism, etc.

3.3.4 Metadata

In both hospitals, the collected data reflected all communication instances, detected breakdown situations, and artifact uses. In Hospital_1, two studies were conducted. Thus, two sets of data were collected – one in January 2008 (Phase 1), and one at the end of the same year (Phase 2). In Hospital_2, one study was carried out in May/June 2009. The total number of data hours and total number of communication events recorded in each study are as follows:

Hopital_1, Phase 1:	79h 40min; 2824 events
Hopital_1, Phase 2:	51h 48min; 2163 events
Hospital_2:	56h 00min; 1738 events

This book is mainly concerned with the results from the analysis of the data subset consisting of all breakdowns. The rest of the communication events recorded were used in several of the quantitative analyses presented, but mostly provided the context in the analysis of breakdowns.

The majority of research questions answered by the results concern the comparison of breakdowns in the two hospitals. Thus, for most of the analyses the data from Phase 1 and Phase 2 are integrated so as to represent the environment of Hospital_1 as a whole. However, the two datasets are considered individually in the context of the technology adoption study, which is concerned with the differences between Phase 1 and Phase 2 in Hospital_1.

3.3.5 Post-data collection coding

The analysis aimed at a thorough understanding of breakdowns by exploring their properties and respective repairs. Information on the types of breakdowns that occur, the types of coordination processes, the types of repair work, and the impact of breakdowns was sought. No previous work was found to define categories for the purpose of examining this kind of information related to breakdowns. Therefore, based on the breakdown and repair properties derived in Chapter 2 on the basis of previous research, and additionally through an iterative process of content analysis of the recorded breakdowns episodes, a coding scheme of breakdown and repair properties was developed for this research. After several cycles of refinement, the scheme was stabilized at the following seven variable categories.

Breakdown type. Breakdowns are classified into four categories – *coordination*, *coordination due to dynamic conditions*, *technical*, and *human errors*. The breakdowns of *coordination* are those that concern the patient care management within and between teams. These breakdowns are preventable, unless they are caused by dynamic conditions. The breakdowns of *coordination due to dynamic conditions* are those that are caused by conditions that are external to the surgical process, *i.e.* breakdowns originating from patients, from hospital bed shortage, staff shortage, etc. *Technical* breakdowns represent unexpected problems with the use of technology of any kind. *Human errors* are related to an individual's cognitive processing of information.

Table 2. Examples of breakdown types.

Type	Breakdown examples observed
Coordination	A porter comes to the Admissions area to take a patient to Holding. However, the patient has not been admitted yet. (Note: Normal coordination of the patient transfer implies that the porter has prior confirmation of the patient having been admitted and assessed by the nurse. Only then should the porter come to take the patient for transfer.)
Coordination due to dynamic conditions	There is a shortage of beds in the inpatient unit. Therefore not all surgical patients scheduled for the day can be admitted, but only those whose procedures would allow them to recover within hours and be discharged the same day (*i.e.* outpatient surgeries). A patient's surgery is cancelled and the order of other scheduled surgeries is rearranged.
Technical	The nurse is unable to check whether the blood tests for her patient are done because the EHR system is down.
Human error	The physician wrote two identical orders for medication to be administered to his eye surgery patient - one order for each eye. The person processing the chart thinks that since the orders are identical, then it must be a duplicate order and throws away one order.

Theme. Content analysis revealed six major themes around which breakdowns occur in the hospitals of this research[1]: *patient care* (related to the process of care), *patient information* (related to the patient chart), *patient status* (location of the patient and/or status of progress of treatment), *contactability* (ability to establish contact with a functional role of interest), *human factors* (slips, lapses and mistakes [238]), and *equipment.*

---

[1] Note that the themes defined here are reflective of the themes identified by other researchers (see Chapter 2), but have been adjusted to better reflect the major clusters of breakdowns that were observed in this study. The 'patient care' theme integrates the issues of surgical schedule, staffing, room assignment, lab services, etc. on the day of surgery. Nevertheless, the specifics of whether the reason for a breakdown was the surgical schedule or another one are recorded in the data and available for the finer-grained analysis. The *patient status* theme includes issues around patient preparedness and around patient location and transfer. *Equipment* breakdowns are as defined by other researchers. The rest of the themes were added to the set as a result of content analysis of the breakdowns data.

Table 3. Examples of breakdown themes.

Theme	Breakdown examples observed
Patient care	▪ Cancellation of surgeries. ▪ Change in the treatment plan.
Patient information	Blood test and/or electrocardiogram (ECG) records in the patient chart are outdated. (Note: records have a validity of three months)
Patient status	▪ The porter is looking for a patient in order to transfer him/her to the next point of care. The patient was already taken by the anesthesia team. ▪ At 10am, the surgeon wants to know whether his scheduled patient for 2:00pm surgery has arrived and been admitted yet.
Contactability	▪ The phone in Holding is ringing and noone is picking it up (staff are either busy or not in the room). ▪ A nurse is paging a surgeon to inform him of his patient's state, which may affect the plan of care. The surgeon is not returning the page.
Human factor	▪ *A slip*: When trying to contact the OR, the nurse mis-dialed the number. ▪ *A lapse*: After completing the patient assessment, the nurse forgot to mark the patient status as "ready" on the board. ▪ *A mistake*: The Admitting nurse completed the patient assessment and transferred the first patient for Dr. X to Holding. She did not realize that even though this was the first patient for Dr. X, the surgery was scheduled for a later time in the day. Patient had to be transferred back to Admission. (Note: first patients are usually scheduled for 8am)
Equipment	▪ There are not enough intravenous (IV) pumps in the Holding area and clinicians need to coordinate the transfer of pumps from other units. ▪ The OR table in the OR is unstable and needs to be fixed.

Tangibility. The property of tangibility measures the role of information salience in breakdowns. In this scheme, two values of tangibility were defined – *tangible* and *intangible*. The tangible represents coordination mechanisms that embed and display information that can be accessed by agents. Tangible mechanisms are relevant to the use of coordinating artifacts such as forms, physical objects, software, etc. where the information about the task at hand is embedded in the artifact, documented for the user, and readily accessible during coordination. Hence, tangible mechanisms relate to information exchanges that are salient and persistent. Breakdowns of this type reflect either failure associated with the use of information that is available through an artifact, or one associated with the improper utilization of an artifact - such as when a form in the patient chart is blank, rather than filled in. Such breakdowns are defined as relating to the tangible.

The intangible represents coordination mechanisms that deal with information that is not salient at the moment of use, nor is it persistent (archival). The breakdowns relating to the intangible occur due to a breakdown in the use of impersonal coordination processes such as protocols, norms, conventions, informal rules, and standards that implicitly carry information used to coordinate the task at hand [280] – i.e. information-discreet mechanisms. Mismatches in clinicians' mental models, or disregard for standards, conventions and protocols, may result in breakdowns related to the intangible.

Table 4. Examples of tangibility.

Tangibility	Breakdown examples observed
Tangible	▪ Blood test records are missing in the patient chart. ▪ Consent form is not signed by the patient and/or the surgeon. ▪ Nurse did not notice a blood test result in the EPR. ▪ The Admission's patient list indicates patientA as being non-infectious, while the OR desk's patient list indicates patientA as being infectious.
Intangible	▪ The whiteboard indicates that patientB is not ready for transfer, but the anesthesia team sends a porter to fetch patientB. (Note: the standard/informal rule is that a porter should only be sent for a patient when the patient is marked as ready by the previous point of care) ▪ Nurse in Holding notices that the patient does not have a signed consent for blood transfusion. The nurse is unsure whether such consent is needed for the particular procedure so she verifies with the surgeon.

Coordination scale. Coordination breakdowns are classified as relevant to *intra-team* coordination (affecting the work within one team), *inter-team* coordination (affecting the work of multiple teams), or both.

Table 5. Examples of breakdown scale.

Scale	Breakdown examples observed
Intra-team	▪ A vitals monitor is not working. The nurse informs the team about the situation. ▪ A team member calls in sick.
Inter-team	The patient consent has not been acquired. The nurse has to arrange that the surgeon comes from the OR to Admission to acquire the patient's consent. Until that has happened the patient's care cannot proceed further to Holding or to the Block Room. (Note: the consent must be signed during a visit to the surgeon's office, in advance of the surgery)
Intra and inter	A patient had consumed water and coffee prior to coming for surgery. The admitting nurse needs to inform the surgeon/anesthetist who will decide when and whether they will proceed with the surgery for this patient. Until that decision is taken the nurse cannot proceed with the patient assessment, nor could the other teams proceed. (Note: Patients are advised not to eat or drink on the morning of their surgery due to risks related to anesthesia)

Breakdown lifetime. Each breakdown is analyzed with respect to its origin, detection location and actual or expected repair location [121] within the macro-surgical system flow represented in Figure 5 and Figure 6. The distance between the three is quantified by a count of the number of micro-systems (micro-system interfaces) between origin-detection-repair. Breakdown lifetime is defined as the total distance between origin and repair. The following example demonstrates the quantification technique in regard to the patient care flow in Hospital_1 (Figure 5):

- Breakdown: unsigned surgery consent form
- Origin: Surgeon's office
- Observed detection: Admission
  - ➢ origin-detection distance = 4
- Repair: OR (contact surgeon in OR to come to Admission and take patient consent)
  - ➢ detection-repair distance = 2
  - ➢ breakdown lifetime = (4 + 2) = 6

Repair strategy. Clinicians resolve breakdowns either through *information pull* (an individual takes the initiative to obtain information of interest) or *information push* (an individual takes the initiative to distribute information to others).

Table 6. Examples of breakdown repair strategy.

Repair strategy	Breakdown examples observed
Information pull	▪ The surgeon notices that a patient's chart indicates outpatient surgery while the surgical schedule indicates inpatient admission for this patient. She calls the OR desk to find out the correct post-operative destination of the patient. ▪ A nurse cannot read the hand-writing of the surgeon for pre-operative medication for the patient. She asks two other nurses to help her read the medication order.
Information push	▪ Nurse calls the OR desk or the surgeon to let them know that the patient consent form is not signed. (Note: the consent must be signed during a visit to the surgeon's office, in advance of the surgery) ▪ A decision is made in the OR that a patient's surgery is changed from inpatient to outpatient. The OR staff notify the OR desk clerk who in turn notifies all teams of the change.

Repair cost. Various metrics can measure the consequences of repair – e.g. monetary cost of human resources devoted to repair and taken from patient care, time spent on fixing a breakdown, number of actions taken as a result of a breakdown, etc. Since this research is concerned with communication, the cost of breakdowns was measured in terms of the number of communication chunks that a breakdown repair incurred. Communication instances such as a telephone call, conversation, note writing, etc. are each defined as a chunk. Thus, if a breakdown repair is achieved by calling someone on the phone and then broadcasting the resolution to one's team, the cost is quantified at 2 communication chunks (1 for the call and 1 for the broadcast).

Table 7. Example of breakdown cost.

Repair cost	Breakdown example observed
3	The surgeon's office missed to order in advance an ECG test for the patient. On the day of surgery the Admission's nurse detects that the ECG is missing from the patient's chart. She checks in the EPR system if the ECG has been ordered and performed and finds that it has not (1 chunk). She pages the ECG contact person (2nd chunk). A minute later ECG staff return her call and they arrange for the ECG to be done (3rd chunk).

The unit of chunk was chosen over that of time (minutes or seconds) because chunks represent a more generalizable unit of measure that transcends the particular instance. In addition, a communication chunk is a more reliable data record because during real-time data collection the observer may have noted the start time of events with a delay.

Interruption. An interruption is a communication event ensuing from breakdown repair efforts that produced a break in the task of an unsuspecting external recipient. An interruption can be mediated by synchronous communication means only – *e.g.* face-to-face or telephone. As part of the *cost* measure, the number of interruptions produced during breakdown repair were counted.

Following content analysis by the researchers, ambiguous breakdown occurrences were discussed with clinical staff until breakdown classification was agreed upon. Nonetheless, some breakdowns could not be classified on all measures because some properties were not applicable. For example, the "repair strategy" could not be determined for a case when a clinician detects a missing form in a patient's chart and does not take any action in response. Also, the "tangibility" could not be determined for cases of human error or for coordination breakdowns triggered by a bed shortage situation in the hospital. Another difficulty in coding a breakdown as per a certain property value related to the fact that on some occasions more than one property value applied to a breakdown. For instance, when a clinician both asks for help upon a breakdown and announces to others that there is a problem, the breakdown repair entails both an information pull and an information push strategy. Table 8 summarizes the properties of breakdowns and repairs that comprise the post-data collection coding scheme, as well as the data sample distribution. The coded breakdowns data is provided in Appendix B.2.

Table 8. Breakdowns and repair properties examined in this study, and their frequencies in the data sample. $N_{(Hospital\_1,\ Phase1)} = 68$. $N_{(Hospital\_1,\ Phase2)} = 166$. $N_{(Hospital\_2)} = 162$. "U = unknown/not applicable/all applicable" - breakdowns for which a value on the given property could not be determined, or multiple values applied.

Property:	Defined by these values:	Frequency/Description		
		Hospital_1		Hospital_2
		Phase1	Phase2	
Breakdown type	coordination coordination due to dynamic conditions technical human error	43 15 7 3	100 39 8 19	98 54 2 8
Breakdown theme	patient care (related to the process of care) patient information patient status (within the care process) contactability (i.e. being reachable) human factors (incl. human errors) equipment	35 11 7 6 5 4	79 17 43 3 17 7	105 27 15 7 5 3
Tangibility of the process related to a breakdown	tangible (information is salient) intangible (e.g. norms and protocols) unknown or both	21 22 U=25	44 36 U=59	35 58 U=69
Coordination scale	intra-team inter-team both (inter- and intra-team) unknown or both	2 38 23 U=5	5 99 56 U=6	15 64 62 U=21
Breakdown lifetime	number of workflow steps between the origin of a breakdown and its repair unknown	Min=0 Max=8 U=2	Min=0 Max=7 U=17	Min=0 Max=5 U=22
Repair strategy	information pull information push unknown or both	26 32 U=10	64 68 U=31	61 50 U=51
Repair cost	amount of communication effort incurred by a repair (e.g. number of phone calls) unknown	Min=0 Max=32 U=3	Min=0 Max=17 U=4	Min=1 Max=34 U=11
Interruption	a communication event, ensuing from breakdown repair efforts, that produced a break in the task of an unsuspecting external recipient	159 Min=0 Max=16		147 Min=0 Max=31

3.3.6 The technology adoption study (Phase 1 & 2 explained)

This book reports a longitudinal observational study that examined the communication issues in the perioperative process of Hospital_1 and their evolution through the introduction of technology. Intensive observations of daily communication behaviors and activities of clinical and administrative staff involved in the surgical process were undertaken in Hospital_1 (Phase 1). The conclusion of the first phase coincided with the start of a hospital initiative to reduce communication between care providers and to increase efficiency. At the time when the first set of observations was completed, the hospital IT department actively involved clinicians in a highly user-centered approach for the design of an application for inter-team communication of patient care status, i.e. an eWhiteboard. The eWhiteboard was to replace patient care coordination via the phone medium. Clinicians were recruited to participate in focus group workshops and to define the information, interaction and functionality requirements. The investigator of this research was invited to participate in the design activities, which she attended and observed. The overall design approach of the eWhiteboard closely conformed to the recommended practices for successful adoption as per recent evolutions of the Technology Acceptance Model (TAM) - user participation, management support, incentive alignment, training, organizational and peer support [284]. The IT department implemented the application as an in-house eWhiteboard that automatically generates the list of patients and physicians for the day. The eWhiteboard also requires clinical staff to update patient status information as they start and complete their care on each surgical patient (Figure 7). The department management supported the initiative and encouraged the participation of clinicians in the design activities. Training and support was provided for clinicians and administrative staff prior to integration into the work processes and thereafter. Eight months after the integration of the eWhiteboard into clinical work an identical second set of observations was carried out (Phase 2).

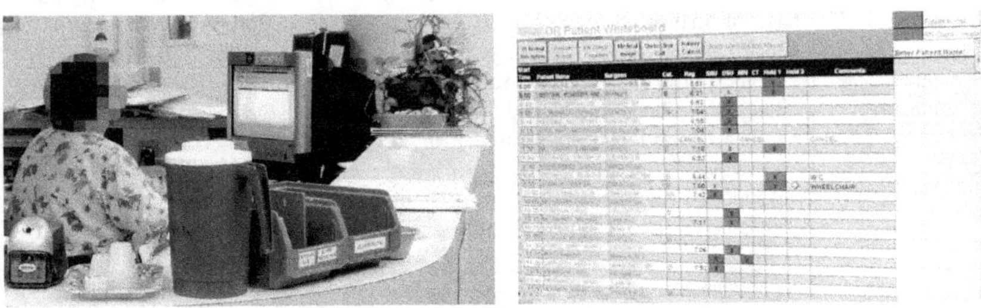

Figure 7: The eWhiteboard. Clinicians checkmark the status of the patient when a patient arrives at the point of care, and when the patient assessment is completed and the patient is ready for handoff to the next point of care.

Participants and data collection procedures in both phases were identical (described in Section 3.3.2). The collected data were complemented with a questionnaire (Appendix A.4) administered after the completion of Phase 2. The questionnaire probed the perception of the utility and satisfaction with the new communication tool. Ten participants returned the questionnaire.

Breakdowns were analyzed post data collection, as described in the previous section. In addition, the specific trigger for a breakdown was considered. Four types of triggers were important for the adoption study: *patient transfer* (related to coordination of patient transfer from one point of care to the next), *awareness* (knowing what is happening), *trust* (a breakdowns triggered by lack of trust in the work of other teams), and *use-error* (a breakdown triggered by an interaction with the eWhiteboard interface). The important breakdown parameters for the adoption study were: *patient status, patient transfer, awareness, trust, use-error, cost, interruptions*. The first three of these – patient status, patient transfer and awareness – were important because the introduction of the eWhiteboard was to coordinate the patient status and transfer by providing awareness. Therefore the eWhiteboard was to eliminate these types of breakdowns. The (lack of) trust and use-errors represent different parameters because they signify specific reasons behind breakdowns. These two particular triggers were introduced into the coding scheme during the analysis of Phase 2 data as it became apparent that the introduction of the eWhiteboard brought about patient status and patient transfer breakdowns that were caused by these factors.

Table 9. Example of adoption study parameters. Patient status is a theme, the remaining parameters are triggers of breakdowns.

Parameter	Breakdown example observed
Patient status	The eWhiteboard indicates that patientC is not admitted yet (*i.e.* the patient has not arrived in the hospital), but the OR desk clerk calls Admissions to confirm that the patient is not there.
Patient transfer	▪ The porter was sent to Admissions to fetch patientD. However, PatientD had already been transferred to Holding by the anesthesia team. ▪ The Block Room requests that three consecutive patients on the schedule for DoctorX be transferred from Admissions to Holding. (Note: There are around 10 doctors, each with a list of scheduled patients for the day. The Holding area and staff can only accommodate one patient per doctor at a time)
Awareness	The Holding area nurse called the Block Room to request information for a patient who had been taken directly to the OR (was not treated at the Block Room). The nurse was not aware the patient was going directly to the OR.
Trust	The eWhiteboard indicates that patientE is in Admissions but is not ready for transfer. The OR desk clerk calls Admissions to confirm that the patient is indeed not ready.
Use-errors	User accidentally selects several patients' entries and updates the status to 'ready', when in fact she meant to update only one patient's status.

It is important to note that in Phase 1, phone calls related to patient status and patient transfer were not considered coordination breakdowns as the phone was the medium facilitating the coordination of the patient care process. However, in Phase 2 the medium was the eWhiteboard. Therefore, phone calls relating to patient status that could have been identified via the eWhiteboard were considered coordination breakdowns.

Table 10 summarizes the breakdown parameters that comprise the post-data collection coding scheme relevant to the technology adoption study as well as the data sample distribution. The data for the adoption study is part of the complete breakdowns dataset provided in Appendix B.2, where Phase 1 or 2 is indicated for each breakdown in the dataset.

Table 10. Breakdowns parameters examined in the adoption study and their frequencies in the data sample. Total breakdowns N = 234 – includes Phase 1 & 2. The frequencies in the table reflect the breakdowns that fell into each parameter category of interest for the adoption study. The rest of the breakdowns are not relevant to the adoption study and therefore not represented in the table.

Category:	Defined by these parameters:	Frequency
Coordination theme	*patient status* - coordination demand within and between teams to establish the status of a patient within the care process	50
Coordination trigger	*patient transfer* - coordination related to the transfer of patients from one point-of-care to another *awareness* - the need to be in the know as to the latest in the status of patient care *trust* – (lack of) trust in the work of other teams *use-error* - whiteboard use related error	15 14 38 10
Consequence	*cost* - amount of communication effort as measured by the number of communication episodes incurred by a repair - e.g. number of phone calls	Min = 0 Max = 32

3.3.7 Safety culture survey

The Safety Attitudes Questionnaire (SAQ) is a survey tool developed to identify teamwork and organizational culture climate factors in healthcare institutions that could negatively affect safety. SAQ has been administered numerous times in the context of OR operations [185, 257]. Through 33 items, the tool measures six dimensions of organizational culture: safety climate, teamwork climate, perceptions of management, stress recognition, job satisfaction and working conditions. Measuring safety culture is one way to proactively identify hospital areas that have an increased chance of experiencing an adverse event and those areas that are rich sources of patient safety best practices. SAQ was developed on the basis of extensive research and validation activities around the world [61, 258].

The SAQ was administered over a web interface available through the

OpenSafety.org website (a non-profit organization committed to enhancing patient safety). A link with the web address was sent out to the surgical division in both hospitals (including nursing, administrative, and other staff) and voluntary anonymous participation was invited. The SAQ questions and the survey results for both hospitals are found in Appendix B.1.

3.3.8 Analysis

In addition to exploratory qualitative analysis carried out throughout the study, a number of other analysis methods were utilized in this research. Observed breakdowns were mapped over the workflow models. This mapping helped graphically capture the trajectories of breakdowns over the work practice. Spearman correlation testing for numerical categories and Chi-square tests for the nominal variables were used to test the hypotheses of association between breakdown properties and repair strategies. Two-sample z-test for proportions at the 95% confidence level was utilized to test for differences between the two hospitals related to the SAQ dimensions, as well as to test for statistical changes in the occurrence of breakdowns before and after technology integration in the adoption study. A t-test for differences in the average cost associated with breakdown repair between the two phases was performed. Regression analysis allowed to describe the relationship between increase in cost and interruptions. Some descriptive statistics were carried out as well.

Initial results were discussed with clinicians and hospital staff and their feedback was used to validate some of the findings.

4

The anatomy of coordination breakdowns: towards understanding breakdowns

This chapter delineates the key findings of the research and discusses critical aspects thereof. It presents an in-depth look into coordination breakdowns acquired through a mixed methods study approach of qualitative and quantitative analysis. Issues of communication technology adoption in the surgical work context are examined as well. The chapter ends with the presentation of two conceptual models: one of breakdowns in the surgical process and one of safety.

The aim of this work is to examine coordination processes and respective breakdowns at a finer level of detail than the high-level concept of coordination, and to derive insights for systems design. The majority of results presented in this chapter are concerned with the comparison of breakdowns in the two hospitals. To that end, the two data sets from the first hospital are integrated to produce a unified picture of the state of breakdowns in that hospital. However, the two datasets are considered individually in the context of the technology adoption study, which is concerned with the differences between Phase 1 and Phase 2 in Hospital_1.

4.1 Two hospitals

This section will examine the similarities and differences between the two hospitals as revealed by a meta-analysis of the recorded breakdowns data and the Safety Attitudes Questionnaire.

4.1.1 Breakdowns overview and comparison

The most breakdowns were detected and repaired at the Admissions area at Hospital_2, while the OR desk was the leading breakdowns arena for Hospital_1. Figure 8 illustrates the average number of breakdowns per hour. The Holding area at Hospital_2 experienced more breakdowns on average than the same area at Hospital_1. However, the average number of breakdowns per hour was comparable at both institutions – thus, the differing averages for each area are reflective of the differing organizational process structures (see Section 3.2.3).

The mean cost associated with a breakdown repair at Hospital_1 and Hospital_2 was compared by means of an independent samples t-test and found consistent between the two datasets (*i.e.* no statistical difference; $t_{(376)}=0.718$; $P=0.473$). Hence, breakdowns produced relatively similar communication overhead in both hospitals.

The average breakdown lifetime (origin-detection-repair distance) was shorter for Hospital_2 – with a mean lifetime of 2.16 micro-systems (*i.e.* process steps) per breakdown, as opposed to 2.86 micro-systems for Hospital_1 ($t_{(342)}=4$; $P<0.001$). The same difference held true for the individual distances of origin-detection ($t_{(351)}=4.5$; $P<0.001$) and detection repair ($t_{(367)}=2.3$; $P=0.023$). The shorter distances at Hospital_2 reflect the more distributed horizontal process structure at that institution and the direct communication lines between micro-systems (see Chapter 3, Section 3.2.3).

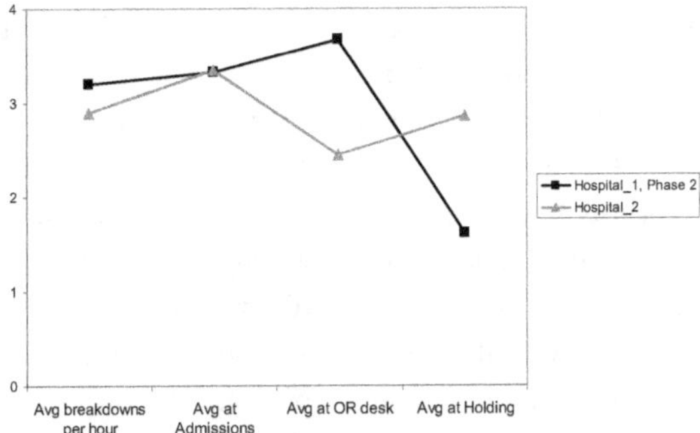

Figure 8: Average number of breakdowns recorded in Hospital_1 and Hospital_2. [2]

The distribution of breakdowns according to the nominal categories of the coding scheme revealed that the types and proportions of breakdowns in the two hospitals were mostly equivalent (Appendix **Error! Reference source not found.**). One difference is that there are significantly more breakdowns due to dynamic conditions at Hospital_2 (P=0.025). This result corresponds logically with the fact that this surgical unit's work is greatly affected by its association with a big trauma centre. The dynamic conditions type of breakdowns also resulted in a greater number of schedule-related breakdowns, though the difference is only significant at the 90% Confidence Interval (P=0.052).

Another difference is that during breakdown repair, information pushing was utilized more at Hospital_1 (P=0.022), while the combination of information push and information pull was utilized more at Hospital_2 (P=0.001) (see Section 4.2.2).

4.1.2 Safety culture

The Safety Attitudes Questionnaire revealed many similar trends and a few differences between Hospital_1 and Hospital_2 (Appendix B.1).

Similarities. Both hospitals' participants rated the *Teamwork Climate* factors to be average, with a notable but non-statistical difference in favor of teamwork at Hospital_2 on the item of cooperation between physicians and nurses ("The physicians and nurses here work together as a well-coordinated team") – 57%

---

[2] The number of hours of observations was the same across Phase 1 and Phase 2 at Hospital_1, and between those and Hospital_2. There was a higher number of recorded breakdowns in Phase 2 and in Hospital_2, which is attributed to the role of learning and conditioning of the observer to greater sensitivity in detecting breakdowns. Therefore, the data averages from Phase 2 of Hospital_1 are considered more representative and comparable to the averages from Hospital_2, and thus are chosen for comparison reasons here.

positive response of clinicians at Hospital_2 as opposed to 35% at Hospital_1.

The *Safety Climate* received average scores for both hospitals as well. In Hospital_1 and in Hospital_2 the ratings for stimuli to report patient safety concerns were high ("I am encouraged by others in this clinical area to report any patient safety concerns I may have") at 71% and 76% respectively. In addition, few respondents were concerned about discussing errors ("In this clinical area, it is difficult to discuss errors") – at 12% and 10% respectively.

Stress Recognition showed that in both hospitals staff were well aware of the effects of stress on performance and consequently on patient safety. One difference in this category emerged on the item for the effects of inter-personal stress ("I am more likely to make errors in tense or hostile situations") where Hospital_2 scored higher recognition of the issue (significant only at the 90% Confidence Interval).

Differences. Statistical significance at the 95% Confidence Interval was found on two of the survey factors: job satisfaction - specifically on the morale dimension (P=0.01); and unit management (P=0.043).

Job satisfaction overall was rated higher by participants from Hospital_1. The statistically significant factor in this category was the issue of morale ("Morale in this clinical area is high"), which was positively rated by 53% of participants from Hospital_1, as opposed to 14% from Hospital_2 (P=0.01). Another strong factor was the perception of the workplace ("This clinical area is a good place to work"), which was rated higher at Hospital_1 (82% at Hospital_1 vs. 52% at Hospital_2) – though significant only at the 90% Confidence Interval.

Perceptions of *Unit Management* were more favorable at Hospital_1 (P=0.043; 71% at Hospital_1 vs. 38% Hospital_2), with the main contributing factor to the high score being the item "Unit management supports my daily efforts".

In summary, the two hospitals exhibited a number of similarities in safety culture. The differences were in Job Satisfaction and Unit Management – in both cases in favor of Hospital_1. There were also two important items with moderate (non-statistical) difference in favor of Hospital_2 – the perception of teamwork between nurses and physicians, and the recognition of the effects of tension and hostile situations on safety.

4.2 Towards understanding breakdowns: qualitative analysis

The amount of effort defines the type of coordination – implicit when coordination work is minimal and explicit when it requires overt articulated effort [181, 256]. Joint activity theory proposes that people follow a least collaborative effort principle [54], i.e. prefer to implicate coordination as much as possible. In Human Computer Interaction these issues have engendered significant research in codifying coordination solutions into widgets, toolkits and frameworks for groupware design that facilitate minimized coordination effort in computer-mediated environments [244].

Exploratory analysis in this work revealed the prominent role of the type of coordination employed – implicit or explicit, and the scale of coordination – inter-team or intra-team, to breakdowns (Figure 9). In this work, implicit coordination is characterized as the utilization of a non-verbal coordination mechanism (*e.g.* a norm), whereas explicit coordination represents the use of verbal communication at the time of coordination. The theoretical construct of implicit coordination includes information distributed in the environment, onto artifacts, and through impersonal coordination means [280] – i.e. standards, conventions, organizational rules, etc.

Type of coordination	**Explicit** (verbal)	**Implicit** (non-verbal)
Coordination scale	**Inter** (multiple teams/micro-systems)	**Intra** (within 1 team/micro-system)

Figure 9: Coordination dimensions.

Coordination occurred in two patterns: clinician-patient and clinician-clinician. Within the clinician-patient scenario, coordination was explicit, standardized, and worked smoothly.

Implicit coordination was employed in the same-time same-place setting only of the clinician-clinician pattern. Contrary to expectations, implicit coordination worked smoothly and created no potential for breakdowns. This can be attributed to the benefits stemming from a shared visual field [315], shared mental model of current conditions [47], and common ground [54].

The clinician-clinician coordination situation consisted of two instantiations – at the intra-team and at the inter-team coordination scale levels. The intra-team coordination consisted mostly of assisting team members with small tasks - *e.g.* with paging someone, ordering blood tests, etc. – through both implicit and explicit means. Intra-team coordination was non-problematic.

Clinician-clinician coordination at the inter-team dimension was explicit and required significant effort, as well as created conditions facilitating breakdowns. Inter-team communication was synchronous or asynchronous, different-place, and mostly mediated. Coordinating artifacts were private objects, rather than shared, and awareness was maintained through an information push/pull approach over the phone medium. The challenge was to stay coordinated across physical spaces and across instances of coordinating artifacts. Coordination breakdowns transpired occasionally and our interviews revealed an overall sense of clinician dissatisfaction with inter-team coordination.

Table 11 describes the observed coordination performance. Next, in Section 4.2.1, the contributing factors behind such performance are analyzed.

Table 11. Observed coordination performance based on four dimensions of communication.

	Implicit	Explicit
Intra-team	good	good
Inter-team	n/a	problematic

4.2.1 Colliding pressures to clinical work

While the information and coordination needs throughout the surgical care process fall within several broad themes (described in Section 4.2.2), the demands and pressures over the work of clinical teams differ across the stages of the process, sometimes in ways that are conflicting, and therefore create latent conditions for inter-team breakdowns. Table 12 shows the pressure points for the major patient care phases in the surgical work process, as observed in Hospital_1 and Hospital_2. Despite the differences in both environments, the pressure points in the two institutions are mostly equivalent in all stages of the care process.

The main pressures in all surgical points of care are often conflicting interests of clinical teams through the patient care stream. Oftentimes these situations arise as a result of changing dynamic conditions such as the emergence of an unscheduled trauma case. Such an emergency case produces the need to re-arrange the surgical schedule – such as delaying or canceling a scheduled surgery due to re-allocation of resources. From a surgeon's perspective (the critical decision maker in this situation), cancellation is a last resort because cancellations increase negative performance metrics and decrease revenue streams. As a result, surgeons push towards keeping scheduled admitted patients, who are 'bumped' by an emergency case and now pending, in the hospital until a possible solution is found for re-including them into the daily operating schedule. From Admission's perspective, holding pending patients in the unit takes hospital beds and ultimately produces a bottleneck where incoming scheduled patients cannot be accommodated. In addition, clinical staff at Admissions would have to interface with pending patients' growing negative experience over the long waiting times and the option of an eventual cancellation of the pending surgery.

Table 12. Work pressure points through the surgical patient care process. "V" = presence of a pressure point.

		Hospital_1	Hospital_2
Admission team	Patients should be prepared on time.	V	V
	Help with work in pre-op holding		V
	Help with work in post-op	V	V
	Patient incompliance (e.g. patient arrives late, patient ate before coming for surgery, etc.)	V	V
	Preparatory work or chart are incomplete	V	V
	Serving as the patients' interface for problems originating beyond Admission (e.g. 2nd cancellation; long waits due to schedule changes)	V	V
	Pressures from down the line (e.g. from OR or Holding)	V	V
	Prioritize patients by schedule vs. by minimizing a surgeon's idle time		V
	Capacity issue – surgeons do not wish to make cancellations, but then Admission reaches capacity and no new patents can be admitted		V
OR desk	Multiple stakeholders' interests, incl. conflicting interests, to be handled and considered	V	V
	Make real-time urgent decisions	(in OR)	V
	Dependence on asset availabilities (e.g. equipment)	(in OR)	V
	Schedule issues (incl. multiple cancellations for the same patient vs. emergency cases - cannot cancel either)	V	V
	Communication overload	V	
	Pressure from OR to get patients earlier	V	
Holding team	Last check point for patients	V	V
	Pressure from OR to get patients earlier ("surgeons should not wait")		V
	Minimize a patient's stay in Holding		V
OR (charge nurse)	Make real-time urgent decisions	V	(in OR desk)
	Dependence on asset availabilities (e.g. equipment)	V	(in OR desk)
	Schedule issues (incl. multiple cancellations for the same patient vs. emergency cases - cannot cancel either)	V	(in OR desk)
Block	Last check point and patient is put under anesthesia	V	V
	Schedule issues vs. patient quality care – anesthesia duration, patient wait time, etc.	V	V
	Make real-time urgent decisions	V	V

The conflicting interests described above demand a great effort in negotiation of plans and re-coordination of actions among multiple stakeholders and teams (*i.e.* at the inter-team level). Further, delayed or cancelled surgeries are associated with a domino effect on the surgical schedule for the day, and consequently on the coordination workload for clinicians, which is a secondary activity to patient care.

Thus, the overall workload and the stress level for clinicians are increased due to the higher demand for coordination and negotiation. In addition to breakdowns related to scheduled patient care, the uncertainty and power dynamics associated with emergencies, unexpected situations, and the need for time-sensitive decisions increase the probability of further coordination breakdowns. For instance, sometimes decisions are made that neglect the current conditions at participating clinical micro-systems and trigger negotiation efforts to modify the decision (as in the above example). Another example is when a stakeholder is accidentally missed in the inter-team coordination effort as in the case of a change in patient order that is not communicated to the Admitting team who begin intravenous medication administration to the now delayed patient due to lack of awareness – an undesirable situation. Hence, there is a combination of high workload, high stress, and high incidence of breakdown repair work, which are exacerbated by colliding micro-systems' pressures. Figure 10 illustrates that breakdowns occur and are dealt with during times of elevated workload - the data represents a typical day shift at the surgical admission units in Hospital_1 and Hospital_2.

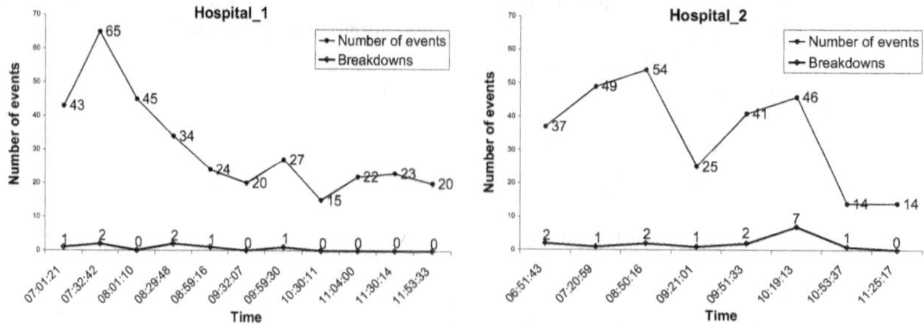

Figure 10: Events and breakdowns during a typical dayshift at the surgical admission unit in Hospital_1 and Hospital_2. The graph shows the cumulative number of communication events over half hour intervals – the graph time span is from 6:30am until 11:53am for Hospital_1, and from 6:17am until 11:25am for Hospital_2. The graph shows that when the workload is high (*i.e.* high total number of events) is also the time when breakdowns are detected and repaired.

The uncertainty as to the status of affairs and consequently the coordination demand are very high, even though coordination should be only a secondary task to patient care. In addition, breakdown repair work generates a number of interruptions to critical primary tasks. For example, in order to make decisions on plans of action related to unanticipated circumstances in planned patient care, clinicians call to speak with the surgeons in the operating rooms. These calls occur while the surgeons are performing operations on patients. The pressure, uncertainty, high workload, and interruptions create the preconditions to human error, communication and coordination breakdowns, and system level breakdowns. These latent factors can potentially result in inadvertent hazards.

4.2.2 Foci of coordination

Coordination occurred around four information foci – patient care, patient status, schedule status and OR status. These focal points uncover that the essential information needs of agents in the surgical activity are related to maintenance of awareness across teams and physical spaces, i.e. macro-system-wide. The foci identify the critical coordination requirements for the perioperative activity.

Patient care: implicit coordination of activity at the intra-team dimension. The plan of care was mediated by the patient chart that followed the patient throughout the surgical journey and contained all medical information needed for surgical care. However, clinicians utilized the chart beyond the medical domain problem space – they had turned it into a coordinating artifact to help them organize their activities. To simplify intra-team coordination, placement of the chart was assigned particular meaning that facilitated implicit coordination and minimized communication effort. Charts placed on the nursing station desk signified those patients who were waiting to be examined. Any nurse could take charge of these patients' care (Figure 11a). Charts placed on a cart indicated that the patients were ready for transfer to the next point of care (Figure 11a). When a patient was examined but required oral medication before transfer, the chart was placed on a special table with the pills taped on top of the chart binder – when the next care provider called for the patient, any available nurse would perform the patient handoff without forgetting to administer the necessary medication (Figure 11b). These observations show that at the intra-team level clinical activity is based on distributing information across the work setting in a way that allows implicit coordination and distribution of patient care among team members with minimal communication cost and without compromising patient safety. These conditions should be explored as requirements for system design.

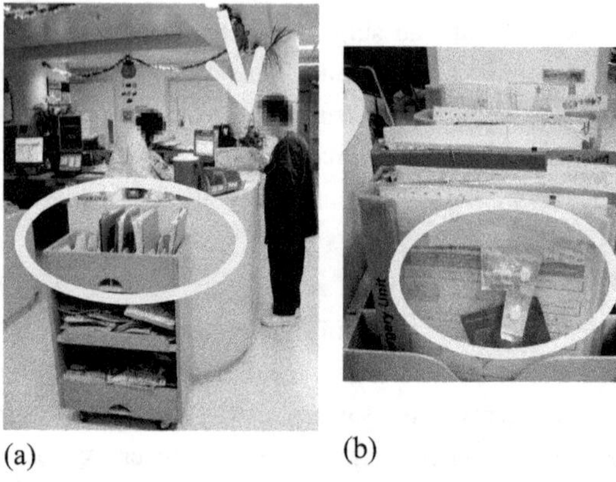

(a) (b)

Figure 11a: A clinician reviews a chart placed on the nursing station desk area for 'patients waiting to be assessed'. The charts on the cart in front of the desk are for patients ready for transfer to the next point of care.

Figure 11b: Medication to be given to the patient upon transfer is visibly placed on top of the patient chart. Any clinician executing the patient handoff can easily learn the patient requires the medication before transfer.

Patient status: the issue of instances of artifacts. Patient status in the process – e.g. location of the patient and progress of treatment at a given point in time – was the most important and difficult coordination issue at the inter-team macro-system level. Locally, intra-team, patient status was established implicitly via a paper artifact listing all the patients scheduled for the day. Due to the differing information needs of teams, each micro-system utilized a unique paper artifact that facilitated patient status identification at the local level. On a macro-system level, there were multiple artifacts targeting patient status information – *e.g.* the Holding Area, the OR desk and the Block Room used schedule printouts from the OR scheduling software – the "OR schedule", while at Reception and Admission a self-devised "Patient List" was utilized in addition to the OR schedule (Table 13). These artifacts were constantly updated with highlights and notes – different types of highlights over patient names indicated that a patient is at the point of care or has been transferred to the next micro-system, a note showed outstanding tests or cancellations, etc. (Figure 12).

Table 13. Coordinating artifacts at each point of care. The artifact types utilized were identical in Hospital_1 and Hospital_2. Each point of care adjusted the presentation of information on the artifacts according to the team information needs, resulting in unique instances of the same type of artifact at each point of care.

	Hospital_1	Hospital_2
Admission team	Patient list OR schedule	Patient list OR schedule
OR desk	OR schedule Emergency list	OR schedule Emergency list
Holding team	OR schedule	OR schedule
OR (charge nurse)	OR schedule Emergency list	OR schedule Emergency list
Block	OR schedule	OR schedule
OR	OR schedule Emergency list	OR schedule Emergency list

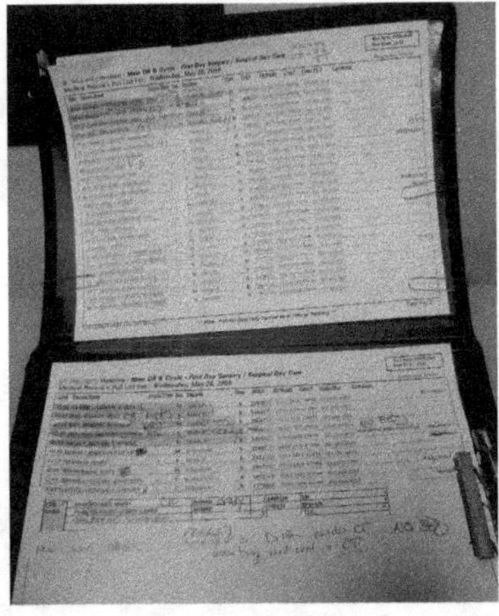

Figure 12: The patient list coordinating artifact. Clinicians mark the status of patients - admitted, being assessed, or transferred, by utilizing different types of highlighting. Notes indicate other important information such as delay of surgery, lack of hospital beds for post-op care, allergies, equipment requirements, etc.

The non-shared patient status information storage resulted in continuous efforts to establish inter-team awareness and align information on artifacts in order to coordinate action (Figure 13). In Hospital_1, the OR clerk's primary role was to mitigate coordination efforts by tracking patient status information, relaying it from one team to another so that teams can coordinate plans and actions. In Hospital_2, clinicians tracked patient status themselves when they needed the information. In both environments, the identification of current patient status was accomplished through a series of phone calls and occasionally through monitoring activity in the immediate surroundings. Inter-team coordination was explicit and associated with a high cost that was additionally exacerbated by the distribution of coordinative efforts across time due to interleaving time-sensitive tasks. Often breakdowns occurred that resulted in further coordination overhead. The challenge of staying aware and coordinated across teams, physical spaces and instances of coordinating artifacts was evident and demands the introduction of mechanisms for facilitation of system-wide real-time patient status awareness.

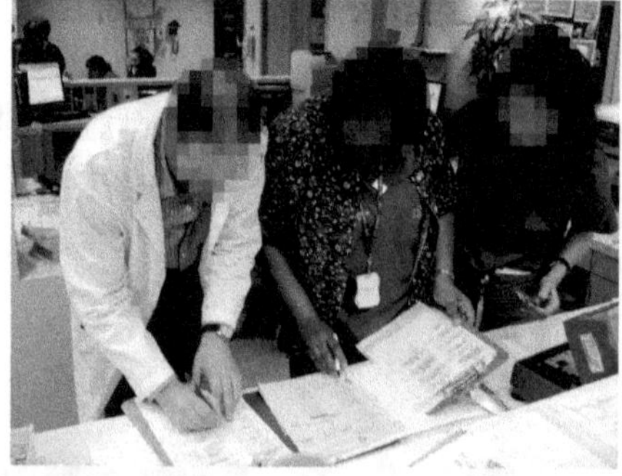

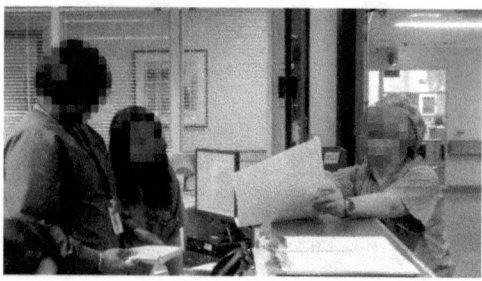

Figure 13: Aligning instances of coordinating artifacts. Clinicians from different teams often have to align information on their instance of the OR schedule, the patient list, or the emergency list, to that of the other teams in order to establish the current status of affairs or to coordinate decisions in regards to schedule changes.

OR schedule status: explicit coordination of patient care. The OR schedule is a representation of the distribution of OR rooms, surgical staff, equipment and scheduled patient procedures. Due to dynamically changing conditions within and outside the hospital (*i.e.* external to the surgical system), the OR schedule is adjusted multiple times throughout the day. Changes are relevant to all participants in the surgical macro-system – local activities and planning at each point of care are determined by the current OR schedule. The schedule status determines the patient care plan at both the intra- and the inter-team dimension.

In Hospital _1, any change to the schedule was first communicated to the OR clerk who broadcasted it through a series of phone calls to all teams – a total of up to 10 information handoffs (Figure 14). For example, if a patient does not show up for surgery, the Receptionist would notify the OR Clerk who, in turn, would notify Admission, Holding, Anesthesia, Block Room, OR, Recovery, Inpatient Units, etc. The OR Clerk documented all changes on his/her local paper instance of the schedule, which was the most up-to-date schedule artifact in the macro-system due to the centralized nature of information distribution in this setting. Clinicians in the immediate surroundings of the clerical area often stepped in to align the information on their instance of the schedule with that of the clerk. The overall culture of communication in Hospital_1 was one of pre-emptively and proactively "pushing" information, achieved through a fomalized centralization of information and a dedicated communication distribution role, *i.e.* the OR clerk.

In Hospital_2, the communication channels for schedule changes were less formalized due to the distributed and more flexible communication structure (Figure 6), as well as the reactive nature of information exchange. A decision for schedule change was broadcast by the decision-making party to the immediately relevant stakeholders only. The remainder of the teams involved received the information upon requesting it, if the need for it arose. For example, if a decision for an emergency case to be taken was made in the OR that would result in a scheduled patient being put on hold or cancelled, the surgeon would coordinate the decision with the anesthesia team and may notify the OR clerk. However, the other teams may or may not be notified, depending on the workload at the OR clerk's desk – they will, however, receive the information if they explicitly request an update on the schedule by calling the OR desk (Figure 14) or the OR. Another consequence of the informal information distribution at Hospital_2 was that a single care provider may receive multiple calls informing her of the same information. Everyone marked the schedule changes when they were informed, similarly to Hospital_1. However, there was not a single instance of the OR schedule artifact that was always up-to-date – the most current instance varied from one moment to the next. The lack of broadcast structure often resulted in breakdowns at the inter-team dimension – a team whose work planning is dependent on the schedule would be left out of the loop of schedule change information distribution. Consequently, clinical work in the 'uninformed' micro-systems would be centered around an expired status of the OR schedule. Eventually, the interdependence of teams would trigger a communication episode between a team that is informed and one that is not. At this point, the breakdown is detected and re-coordination effort begins. For example, a patient called Admissions to cancel her surgery. Admissions noted the cancellation on their instance of the OR schedule but did not inform other stakeholders. When the time for the patient's surgery approached, Holding called Admissions to request that the patient be transferred – at this point it became known to Holding that this surgery was cancelled. Since the next patient on the schedule for that particular OR was not ready, the consequence of this breakdown was that the OR had to be put on hold until the next patient was ready – with the physicians, nurses and anesthetists waiting. In the context of the perioperative setting, this represents a breakdown with a major impact. Not only does it increase the overall stress level, but it triggers the domino effect on the daily schedule that results in further cancellations, breakdowns, and loss of revenue. The overall culture of communication in Hospital_2 can be characterized as one of "pulling" information per need.

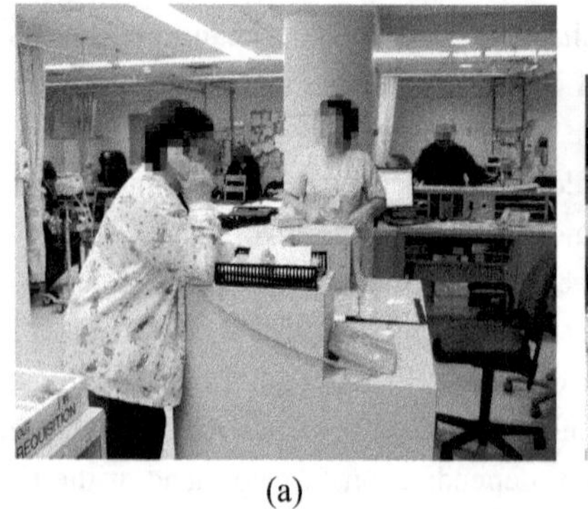

(a)

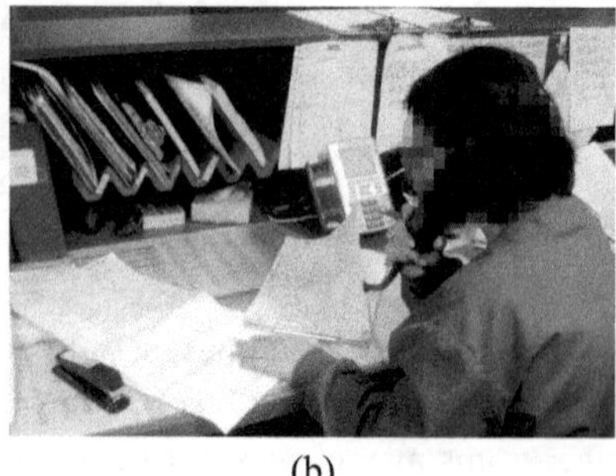

(b)

Figure 14a: Clinician speaking on the phone to the OR clerk regarding a schedule change.

Figure 14b: The clerk gathers and distributes patient care and schedule information through the phone medium and updates the status by marking her instance of the OR list.

The two differing situations described above are strong evidence of the need for real-time information diffusion across the entire socio-technical macro-system, as it is critical to maintain awareness system-wide in order to align plans for patient care. Essentially, implicating inter-team coordination related to scheduling is deemed advantageous.

OR status: the issue of coordination over the wall. Early completion of surgical procedures, as well as complications during surgery and respective delays, affect the OR schedule, patient care and work planning for all teams. In addition, some types of anesthesia administered to a patient in the Block Room require closely-coupled coordination based upon the progress of ongoing surgery in the OR. Inter-team coordination with ORs is critical to safety, but is challenging as it is secondary focus to the OR team – the primary task is performing surgery on their present patient. In addition, most of the OR team members need to maintain sterility which precludes them from using the phone or intercom – they would have to relay the information to a non-sterile nurse who will communicate it externally to other teams. This chain of communication imposes additional inter-team coordination costs. To minimize it, clinicians from teams outside the operating rooms would walk into the ORs to discuss or clarify important OR status information. They fought the communication constraints of distributed physical spaces by creating an opportunity for synchronous same-place communication for successful coordination of action. This finding is in sync with Coiera's observation that clinicians have a synchronous bias and favor information seeking from humans [59]. However, such practice can be a threat to safety as it introduces interruptions and additional cognitive demands to OR staff. Thus, there is a need for surgical procedure progress awareness mechanisms that distribute information on the state of affairs inside the operating room so that the coordination needs of non-OR staff are met without risking patient safety. This finding adds further evidence for the requirement to maintain system-wide awareness.

4.2.3 Recurrent patterns of coordination

Recurrent breakdowns are repeated situations when staying coordinated among agents in the socio-technical macro-system is challenged and the result is loss of common ground, or of shared understanding of the state of the system. Such recurrent problems of coordination trigger the creation of coordination structures, either in the form of conventions or as formal procedures, to mitigate coordination efforts. Since these structures of coordination are consistently used to solve the same coordination problem, they are referred to as *patterns*. The coordination patterns observed aimed at avoiding safety threats and the occurrence of breakdowns. The patterns were, however, cumbersome communication structures – often producing interruptions to clinical work, ambient noise in an already hectic environment, and adding to the cognitive load of participants. Nonetheless, the patterns of coordination are important because they reveal the critical communication needs and requirements of clinicians in coordinating their daily work.

In Hospital_1, the observations revealed several coordination patterns devised by hospital staff to facilitate the recurrent problems of coordination and maintenance of awareness. The use of these structures was consistent and was confirmed through informal interviews. Formalized descriptions are presented in Figure 15. In Hospital_2, only one pattern was observed. As mentioned earlier, the culture of communication at this institution was more flexible and reactive in nature, which explains the less formalized ways of coordination. The following discussion on patterns of coordination is based on the study from Hospital_1.

One pattern utilized at the Reception and Admission areas related to inter-team coordination of patient transfer to the next point of care, which required establishing patient status within the immediate environment - e.g. whether the patient has arrived, has been brought in, has been assessed, or needs medication administration. The structure of action sequences is presented in Figure 15, Pattern 1. The sequence demonstrates the desire for least coordinative effort – implicit coordination is empowered via chart placement, and explicit coordination is only a backup strategy. The structure also allows distribution of responsibility for inter-team coordination in an implicit manner across all local team members – i.e. any clinician can establish patient status to coordinate patient transfer.

The OR Clerk's function was the most demanding in terms of frequency and density of coordination tasks. The schedule-related broadcasting structure to maintain inter-team awareness consisted of multiple steps (Figure 15, Pattern 2) and required a high level of cognitive load due to numerous interruptions and parallel tasks. For example, a broadcast could span over 15 minutes and 20 recorded communication events – where only 6 of the events were related to the broadcast structure instance.

Implicit structures were devised where appropriate to reduce task load for the OR clerk and to allow redistribution of cognitive resources to other explication-demanding coordinative tasks. Figure 15, Pattern 3 shows the way paper slips mediated coordination of patient transfer between the OR Clerk and the Attendants. Similar to Pattern 1, this structure implicitly distributed the coordination throughout the socio-technical system. The structure was embedded within the ongoing task of maintaining awareness – i.e. both the clerk and attendant integrated the new information onto their individual coordinating artifacts – so that they can plan their activities based on current state of affairs.

Pattern 1:
Establish patient status to coordinate inter-team transfer

```
<look for placement of chart in "ready" spot>
if chart is NOT in a "ready" spot:
    <look at patient list markings>
    if markings are insufficient:
      <look around & inquire team members>
    end if
end if
if medications are taped on chart
    <give medications to patient>
end if
```

Pattern 2:
OR Clerk broadcasts schedule change

```
for all to whom this is relevant:
   <call Admission>
   <call Holding>
   <call OR>
   <call Block Room>
   <call Recovery>
   <call Inpatient Units>
   <tell porter>
   <page Charge Nurse>
   <take call from Charge Nurse>
```

Pattern 3:
OR clerk coordinating patient transfer with Attendant

```
<mark OR list when call for patient is done>
<take patient slip from "hold" location>
<tape patient slip to front of desk>
Attendant:
    <take patient slip>
    <cross check patient info against OR schedule>
    <go for the patient>
if attendant is back & takes a blanket:
    <highlight patient name on OR schedule as "arrived">
end if
```

Figure 15: Patterns of coordination in Hospital_1.

4.2.4 Summary of qualitative findings

The qualitative analysis resulted in a few major findings. First, it identified that perioperative work at the intra-team coordination dimension is realized smoothly – both through implicit and explicit means. Significant effort and potential for breakdowns were observed with inter-team coordination that was explicit. The challenges contributing to the problematic inter-team coordination were: 1) colliding pressures between micro-systems, 2) maintaining awareness of the state of affairs by having to align multiple instances of coordinating artifacts, 3) the effects of dynamically changing conditions on intra- and inter-team patient care planning, and 4) coordination of tightly-coupled actions among teams in separate physical spaces. Finally, in Hospital_1, several patterns of coordination were observed as solutions devised by clinicians to solve recurrent coordination breakdown situation.

The findings contradict common beliefs of implicit coordination being a safety issue and reveal that breaks in continuity of surgical patient care occur mostly at micro-system boundaries. These insights are informative of the underlying coordination problems in the surgical process, but cannot adequately describe the severity of the breakdowns that occur. To that end, further investigation of breakdowns was conducted with a quantitative approach.

4.3 Quantitative analysis

In order to examine the hypotheses defined in Chapter 2, Section 2.4, as well as to determine the severity of breakdowns identified through the qualitative approach, statistical measures were applied to the data from both Hospital_1 and Hospital_2. In this section, the origins and lifetimes of breakdowns are dissected. The role of tangibility of broken coordination mechanisms is examined, and its relation to other properties of breakdowns and repairs. Also, the determinants of the choice for breakdown repair strategy are investigated. Lastly, the breakdown properties that determine breakdown impact and repair costs are explored.

The results presented in this section are concerned with the comparison of breakdowns in the two hospitals. To that end, the two data sets from Hospital_1 are integrated so as to represent the environment of Hospital_1 as a whole. In the next section (Section 4.4), the two datasets from Hospital_1 are considered individually and are juxtaposed in order to examine the problem of technology adoption and occurrence of breakdowns.

The following results are derived from the coded breakdowns data (Appendix B.2). Breakdowns are analyzed statistically according to each property they were coded by (*e.g.* breakdowns scale) and hypotheses are tested for the relation between two distinct properties of the same breakdown (*e.g.* breakdown scale and tangibility). For each statistical test, the breakdowns that did not have a value for the properties tested were excluded.

4.3.1 Propagation of breakdowns

Breakdowns originate throughout the perioperative process. The initial trajectory of breakdowns, as determined by whether they were detected at origin or not, is shown in Figure 16. Our results reveal that most breakdowns propagate downstream in the surgical system flow and therefore affect perioperative work downstream, i.e. at the inter-team dimension. The degree of propagation is significant - what Figure 16 reveals is that 86% and 88% of all breakdowns with an identifiable origin propagated downstream in Hospital_1 and Hospital_2, respectively.

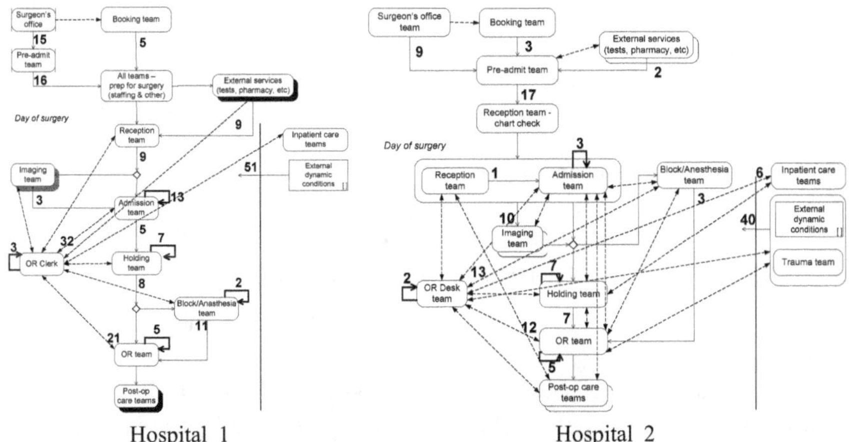

Figure 16: Breakdowns propagation. The numbers represent the count of breakdowns originating from each micro-system. A loop indicates a breakdown detected at origin. Communication lines without associated number next to them indicate that no breakdowns on those pathways were observed during the study. Most breakdowns propagate downstream or through the communication channels upstream, i.e. breakdowns are mostly at the inter-team level.

Breakdown content analysis through the *coordination scale* property confirmed that the majority of breakdowns relate to inter-team coordination processes (Figure 17). In fact, given that the "inter and intra" category value is defined as breakdowns that affected both intra- and inter-team processes, we could conclude that 97% of breakdowns in Hospital_1 affected inter-team work, and respectively 89% of breakdowns in Hospital_2.

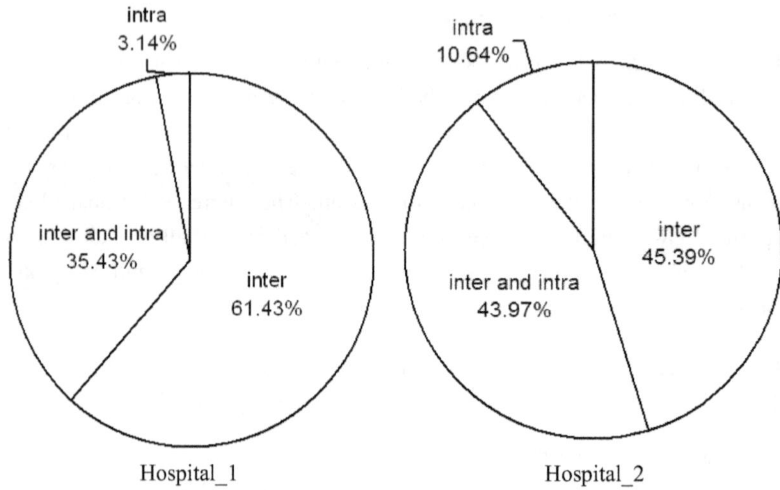

Figure 17: Relevance of breakdowns to scale of coordination.

4.3.2 Tangibility of coordination and breakdowns

Hypothesis 1: Tangibility of coordination mechanism relates to breakdown theme.

An association between tangibility and breakdown theme was found in both hospital settings (P<0.001 in Hospital_1 and in Hospital_2, Chi-Square exact test). Examination of the Adjusted Standardized Residuals (

Table 14) showed that the major contributing factors in the association were the following themes:

- Hospital_1: human factors, patient information, patient status, and equipment
- Hospital_2: patient information, patient status and patient care

The common contributing themes between the two hospitals were patient information and patient status. Most patient information breakdowns were related to the tangible – to the use of paper forms, software and other artifacts (85.7% and 85.2% in each hospital respectively). The vast majority of patient status breakdowns, on the other hand, were related to the intangible – i.e. to the norms and conventions of practice at the unit (97.9% and 100% for each hospital respectively).

Table 14. Breakdown themes as contributing factors to the association with tangibility of coordination. The adjusted standardized residual indicates the strength of association for each theme - a value equal to or above 2.0 is statistically significant. The higher the value, the stronger the statistical association. Themes in bold indicate significance in both hospitals. Non-significance is indicated by "n.s.".

Breakdown theme associated with tangibility	Adjusted Standardized Residual Hospital_1	Hospital_2
patient care	n.s.	3.7
patient information	**4.9**	**6.0**
patient status	**7.1**	**3.0**
contactability	n.s.	n.s.
human factors	4.4	n.s.
equipment	2.3	n.s.

The remainder of the breakdown themes did not exhibit a common degree of statistical strength across the two hospitals. Nevertheless, it is worth noting the non-statistical commonalities observed. Most human factors based breakdowns (94.1% and 66.7% in each hospital respectively) were related to the use of artifacts, i.e. to the tangible. All equipment breakdowns (100%) were also related to the tangible. The majority of patient care breakdowns (60.8% and 79.6% in each hospital respectively) were related to the intangible. For instance, when surgeons switched ORs but did not notify the Block Room, clinicians in the Block Room were confused to find that the OR they were planning to take patientX to was occupied by another surgeon (from the one they expected in that OR) who was operating on another patient. Finally, all contactability breakdowns (100%) were due to cultural norms - i.e. the intangible. For example, paging surgeons from Admission would get no response as the surgeon does not recognize the caller number. However, paging him/her from the OR Clerk's extension receives timely response as this extension is known as the "OR number" and therefore as an important one.

Hypothesis 2: Tangibility of coordination processes relates to coordination scale (inter, intra, or both).

No relationship of association was found ($P=0.163$ for Hospital_1 and $P=0.285$ for Hospital_2; Chi-Square exact test).

Hypothesis 3: Tangibility of coordination processes relates to the type of repair strategy employed.

Statistical association was found between these two categories ($P<0.001$ for Hospital_1 and $P=0.019$ for Hospital_2; Chi-Square exact test). The Adjusted

Standardized Residuals for information pull and information push were significant for both datasets - 4.8 in the case of Hospital_1, and 2.4 in the case of Hospital_2. From the tangible-based breakdowns 67.3% (Hospital_1) and 52% (Hospital_2) were repaired by information push, and the rest by information pull. From the intangible-based breakdowns, 76% (Hospital_1) and 77% (Hospital_2) were repaired via information pull and the rest via information push.

4.3.3 Repair strategies

Clinicians and administrators work hard to minimize the effects of breakdowns in an effort to preserve the safety and reliability of the system. Thus, each breakdown is associated with a repair that aims to bring the state of processes to what is considered a normal operational state. Repairs are consequential to breakdowns and therefore are expected to be related to breakdowns.

Hypothesis 4: Breakdown type relates to repair strategy.

In Hospital_1, there was an association between the type of breakdowns – coordination, coordination due to dynamic conditions, technical or human error – and repair strategy ($P<0.001$; Chi-Square exact test). The Adjusted Standardized Residuals revealed that the statistical significance comes from the categories of coordination, and coordination due to dynamic conditions (Adj Std Residuals = 4.0 and 3.8, respectively). Coordination breakdowns were resolved with information pull in 59% of cases within this measure, while coordination breakdowns due to dynamic conditions were resolved with information push in 76% within this measure.

In Hospital_2 this hypothesis was not confirmed ($P=0.289$; Chi-Square exact test). Examining the Adjusted Standardized Residuals, however, pointed to similar tendencies as in Hospital_1: coordination breakdowns were resolved with information pull in 56.9% of cases within this measure.

Hypothesis 5: Breakdown theme relates to repair strategy.

An association between breakdown theme and repair strategy employed was found ($P<0.001$ for Hospital_1 and $P=0.002$ for Hospital_2, Chi-Square exact test). As can be seen in Figure 18, most values in the category breakdown theme have a bias in repair strategy (*i.e.* more than 60% of cases). In Hospital_1, contactability, equipment, patient care and patient information related breakdowns are rectified mostly through information pushing, while the majority of breakdowns linked to patient status and human factors are repaired through information pulling. For example, patient status breakdowns are usually related to lack of mutual organizational awareness, and are dealt with by pulling information, i.e. inquiring about the patient status. A review of the Adjusted Standardized Residuals revealed that the statistical significance comes from the patient care, patient information and patient status breakdowns (Adj Std Residuals = 4.1, 3.7 and 7.8, respectively).

In Hospital_2, a similar trend is observed – equipment and patient information breakdowns are resolved through the means of information pushing, while human factor and patient status breakdowns through information pulling. However, the Adjusted Standardized Residuals showed that the statistical significance is mostly due to the patient status breakdown theme (Adj Std Residual = 3.2).

The theme with a common bias between Hospital_1 and Hospital_2 is that of patient status. Although not statistically significant, biases in repair strategy were observed for both hospitals for the other breakdown themes as well.

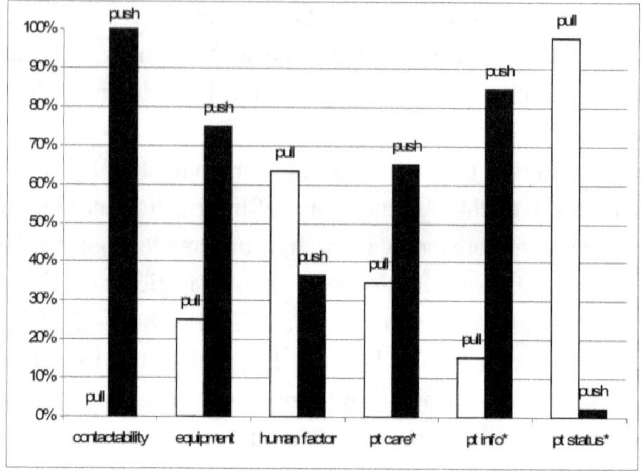

Hospital_1

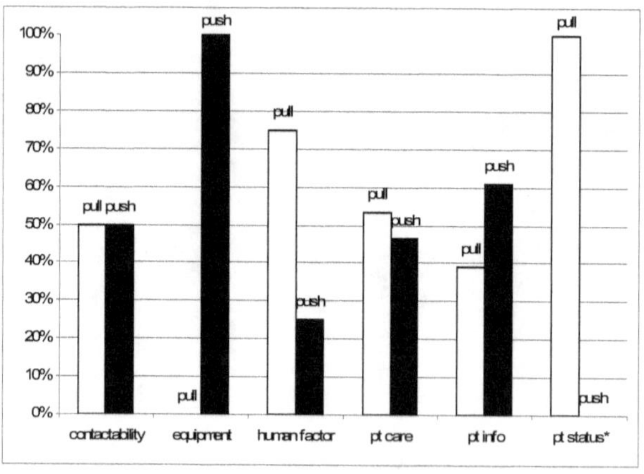

Hospital_2

Figure 18: Breakdown themes and repair strategies (black = information push; white = information pull). A star (*) indicates statistical significance.

4.3.4 Breakdown cost: communication overhead

The number of communication chunks associated with repair from a breakdown reflects the degree of communication overhead that a breakdown induces, and is therefore defined as the repair cost.

Hypothesis 6: Breakdown lifetime (origin-detection-repair) correlates with repair cost.

We found that breakdown lifetime is a predictor of repair cost (P<0.001 for both hospitals; Spearman's rho=0.596 for Hospital_1; Spearman's rho=0.466 for Hospital_2). The same relationship was found between the origin-detection distance and repair cost; as well as between the detection-repair distance and repair cost. The positive correlation indicates that the longer a breakdown propagates downstream in the system process, the greater the communication overhead associated with the repair will be. Propagation ranged from 0 to 4 surgical flow micro-systems. Breakdown cost ranged from 0 to 32 communication chunks per breakdown for Hospital_1 and from 0 to 34 chunks for Hospital_2, with an average of 4 chunks in either case. Figure 19 shows that increase in lifetime tends to result in increase in repair cost.

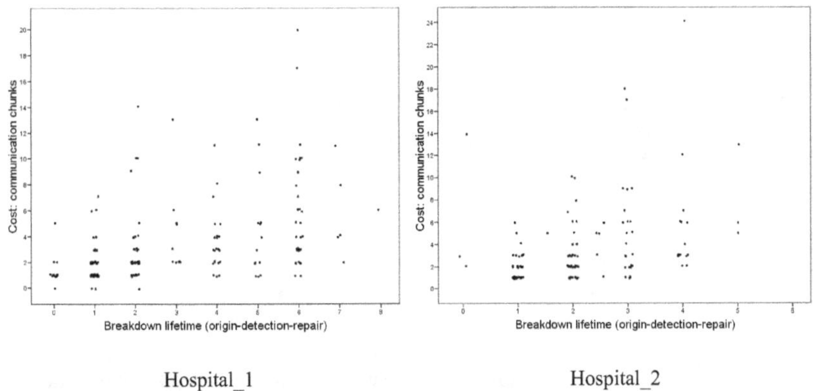

Figure 19: Breakdown lifetime (cumulative distance between origin-detection-repair locations) vs. repair cost, $N_{(Hospital\_1)}$=214 and $N_{(Hospital\_2)}$=135. A random number between -0.1 and +0.1 was added to each discrete measure to facilitate the display of all data points. The graph shows a general increase in distance is associated with increase in cost.

4.3.5 Breakdown cost: interruptions

A significant correlation was found between the *cost* of a breakdown and the number of *interruptions* associated with the repair (Pearson r = 0.948)[3].

[3] The statistic presented is for the combined data from Hospital_1 and Hospital_2. The relationship for the individual hospital data sets exhibited the same correlation.

Regression analysis showed that the model was with predictive power (R^2= 0.898) and the overall relationship was statistically significant (P<0.001). The amount of interruptions as a result of a breakdown can be predicted by the formula:

$$interruptions = 0.796 \times cost - 0.120 \qquad \text{(Eq. 1)}$$

In other words, 68% of communication cost associated with a breakdown repair can be predicted to be interruptive in nature. The mean repair cost across all breakdowns was 3.44 communication chunks. Figure 20 shows the relationship between repair cost and interruptions.

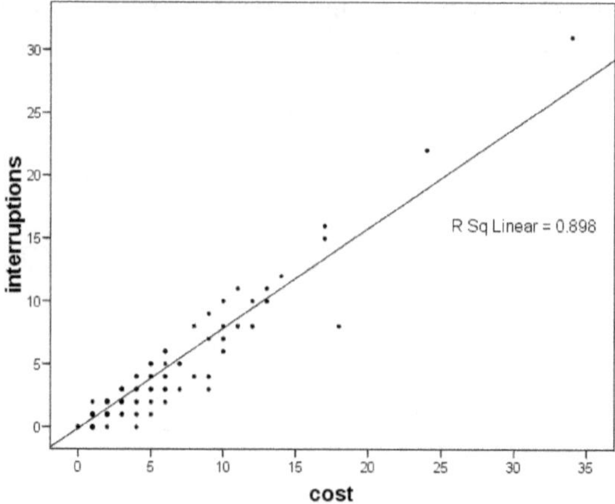

Figure 20: The relationship between breakdown repair cost and the number of interruptions generated.

4.3.6 Breakdown cost: safety

High cost breakdowns for the two hospitals were examined – the top 10% in terms of the number of communication chunks incurred during repair (Table 15). Each breakdown from the data subsets for both hospitals was flagged if it exhibited reasonable potential for a patient safety threat. For example, the following breakdown records were determined as safety-threatening:

- "*unclear pt destination of an add-on case causes great confusion and repair work to clarify if everyone is aware that this pt is having surgery today*".
- "*significant OR delay due to wrong booking - consent was right but surgery booked wrong; could have performed different surgery...*"

All high-cost breakdowns, with only one exception, were of the breakdown type *coordination* (N=15) or *coordination due to dynamic conditions* (N=20) – *i.e.* 35

out of the 36 breakdowns. Statistical difference between the two hospitals was found in the amount of safety-threatening breakdowns (P=0.014; 95% Confidence Interval). In Hospital_2, breakdowns with the highest cost were strongly correlated with safety – 5 out of the 14 breakdowns were patient safety threats as well. This was unlike Hospital_1, where only 1 out of the 22 breakdowns presented a safety hazard.

Table 15. Data subset with top 10% highest cost breakdowns.

	N	Top 10% cost range
Hospital_1	22	Min = 9 Max = 32
Hospital_2	14	Min = 8 Max = 34

4.3.7 Summary of quantitative findings

Breakdowns originate throughout the surgical macro-system (i.e. in all micro systems), and they are rarely rectified at the point of origin – breakdowns propagate downstream in the surgical system in 86% of cases at Hospital_1 and 88% of cases in Hospital_2. A consequence of breakdown propagation is that the majority of breakdowns are related to and affect inter-team coordination – they are found at communication interfaces between micro-systems. Most importantly, the distance a breakdown propagates through the surgical process before being resolved (i.e. from originating point of care to the point of detection and repair) correlates to the breakdown repair cost. Further, 68% of the repair cost of a breakdown is made up of interruptions to ongoing clinical care tasks. The majority of high-cost (top 10%) breakdowns in this study were either of type *coordination* or of type *coordination due to dynamic conditions.*

The breakdown theme relates to the tangibility of the broken coordination process. The common theme predictors between the two surgical units were that of patient information and patient status. Patient information breakdowns related to the tangible - patient information is saliently stored on hard or soft storage media throughout instances of medical environments. Patient status breakdowns, on the other hand, were associated with cultural norms, i.e. the intangible norms and conventions of the local work practice.

The type of repair strategy employed is determined by a combination of the tangibility and theme associated with a breakdown. Tangible-related breakdowns tend to be repaired through information push while normative intangible-based ones tend to require information pull for repair. The breakdown theme also determines the repair strategy to be employed. Across the two hospitals, patient status breakdowns were repaired with information pull. Further, in Hospital_1, patient information and patient care breakdowns exhibited a preference for an information push repair. Although not statistically significant, biases in repair strategy were observed for the other breakdown themes as well.

One interesting difference between the two surgical units' recorded activities was that the highest costing breakdowns were imposing safety threats at Hospital _2, which was not the case at Hospital_1.

Table 16 summarizes the findings.

Table 16. Quantitative results. Findings in bold highlight positive results common to both hospitals.

Finding	Hospital_1	Hospital_2
Breakdowns originate throughout the process and propagate downstream.	True 86%	True 88%
Most breakdowns relate to inter-team coordination	True 97%	True 89%
Tangibility of coordination process relates to breakdown theme.	True $P<0.001$; $\chi 2$ exact test	True $P<0.001$; $\chi 2$ exact test
Tangibility of coordination process relates to coordination scale.	No $P=0.163$; $\chi 2$ exact test	No $P=0.285$; $\chi 2$ exact test
Tangibility of coordination process relates to repair strategy.	True $P<0.001$; $\chi 2$ exact test	True $P=0.019$; $\chi 2$ exact test
Breakdown type relates to repair strategy.	True $P<0.001$; $\chi 2$ exact test	No $P=0.289$; $\chi 2$ exact test
Breakdown theme relates to repair strategy.	True $P<0.001$; $\chi 2$ exact test	True $P=0.002$; $\chi 2$ exact test
Breakdown lifetime relates to repair cost.	True $P<0.001$; rho=0.596	True $P<0.001$; rho=0.466
Breakdowns produce interruptions.	True (68% of cost is interruptions) Pearson $R = 0.948$; $P<0.001$; $R^2=0.898$ interruptions = 0.796 x cost – 0.120	
Big breakdowns threaten safety.	No	True

4.4 Adoption and breakdowns

Many of the breakdowns that emerged during this study's analyses were related to the use of paper artifacts as a medium for the coordination of clinical activity. An intuitive progression of the identification of such artifacts as problematic is to replace them with electronic solutions. An investigation of the adoption of such an electronic solution was conducted before (Phase 1) and after (Phase 2) technology implementation in Hospital_1 (as described in Section 3.3.6). This analysis was conducted to capture the changes in communication and coordination practices resulting from the introduction of the technology. This section describes the findings related to the eWhiteboard communication technology integration into the surgical unit's work. The chapter identifies some socio-cultural factors that underlie the presence of continuous breakdowns in clinical work.

In this section the two datasets (Phase 1 & Phase 2) from Hospital_1 are considered individually and are juxtaposed in order to examine the problem of technology adoption and occurrence of breakdowns. The results presented are derived from the raw data and the coded breakdowns data (Appendix B.2), excluding the breakdowns for Hospital_2. The statistical analysis is provided in Appendix B.5.

Communication Load. Eight months after the integration of the eWhiteboard, the communication workload was reduced from 61 to 42 communication episodes per hour on average for all surgical care areas. The most significant reduction was observed in the work of the OR desk – a decrease of 27 communication episodes per hour, and the least in the work of the Admission team – a decrease of 13 episodes per hour (Table 17).

Table 17. Number of communication episodes per hour comprising patient care work before and after the introduction of the eWhiteboard. Total communication episodes: $N_{(Phase\ 1)} = 2824$ and $N_{(Phase\ 2)} = 2163$.

	Number of communication episodes		
Care Team	**Phase 1 (before)**	**Phase 2 (after)**	**Difference**
Admission	70	58	-13
OR desk	66	39	-27
Holding	43	19	-23
All teams	61	42	-19

Qualitative observations. From the first day of observations in the second phase, it became obvious that patient status-related phone calls were still happening at least several times a day, though reduced in number. The situation was associated with dissatisfaction from those on the receiving end of the calls. The qualitative analysis of participants' comments during observation times revealed that the persisting phone calls in Phase 2 are triggered by lack of trust in the work of other humans - specifically, the lack of trust was exhibited at micro-system boundaries, *i.e.* between points of care. For example, a person from TeamX would state that a patient must have been admitted despite the fact that the eWhiteboard indicates the opposite. The reasoning provided was that the Admission team must have forgotten to update the status or did not know how to update the status. As a result, that person would place a phone call regarding the status of the respective patient. Table 18 lists several snippets from our data log comments that show dissatisfaction on the part of those 'distrusted' and on the part of those who 'do not trust'.

Table 18. Comments and observer notes from the observations log of Phase 2.

Observer note:	"Porter came to get patient who is not here yet, so whiteboard is not honored. ..... patient was clocked-in at Reception but not at Admission yet. ...... A lot of dissatisfaction expressed with dishonoring the whiteboard info. Dissatisfaction with inter-team work"
Observer note:	"unhappy with the pre-admit/prep work- with orders marked 'done' when they were just 'scheduled'"
Participant:	"this is the third time they are calling for this patient"
Observer note:	"[OR clerk checks whiteboard and calls X team]. [X] went to check everything with clerk on hold. Unwarranted – pt not ready, as was marked on whiteboard"
Observer note:	"[OR calls for a patient]. X frustrated coz they call 10 times for same patient"
Observer note:	"[call to Admission team] Confirming that the patient is ready. The whiteboard says 'ready'"
Observer note:	"[X] says she thinks that nurse in [Y team] probably didn't check at the right place to find patient. [X] will call." "they were unhappy. They asked if she looked at the whiteboard. Patient is not in [Y team area] yet and the whiteboard says so." three minutes later: "patient is now marked as 'arrived' on the whiteboard. She makes a remark about the patient being there few seconds later – thus, he must have been there [before]"
Participant:	"why are they not thinking?"
Observer note:	"[X] updates the whiteboard and calls again to tell [Y team] about the switching and to check the whiteboard [about it]. They say they saw it"

Breakdowns. As expected, breakdowns related to *awareness* were significantly reduced after the introduction of the eWhiteboard, from 27% to 2.9% ($P<0.001$). However, contrary to expectations, *patient transfer* related breakdowns slightly increased, rather than decreased, from 5.4% to 9.6%. The increase was not statistically significant ($P=0.211$) and therefore no change is concluded. The average cost of a *patient transfer* breakdown was 1.67 communication episodes. A statistically significant increase in the *patient status* related breakdowns was observed ($P=0.007$). The lack of *trust* in others' work and whiteboard-related *use-errors* accounted for this increase. These two types of breakdown triggers were new and unique to Phase 2. Lack of *trust* produced 72.9% of all patient status coordination breakdowns in the second phase, or 27.9% of all breakdowns with an identifiable trigger in that phase. A total of 35 phone calls were observed in Phase 2 triggered by patient status inquiries despite the whiteboard presence (such phone calls were not considered breakdowns in Phase 1). In 80% of these calls, the status was accurately displayed on the whiteboard. *Use-errors* associated with the eWhiteboard generated another 7.4% of all breakdowns in Phase 2. The average cost associated with *trust*-related breakdowns was 1.5 communication chunks, and that of use-errors was 1.22 chunks. These results are presented in Table 19 and Appendix B.5.

An independent samples t-test was conducted to compare the breakdown repair costs in Phase 1 and Phase 2. The results showed that the average repair cost was consistent across both phases, i.e. no significant difference was found ($t_{(84)}$=1.756; P=0.083).

Table 19. Patient transfer and patient status change from Phase 1 to Phase 2, and the average cost of a breakdown repair across both phases.

Parameter:	Change:	Avg. cost
patient transfer	non-significant increase (P = 0.211)	1.67
patient status →of those, due to trust	increase (P = 0.007) +72.9%	1.56
awareness	significant decrease (P < 0.001)	2.15
trust use-errors	+27.9% +7.4%	1.5 1.22

Perceived usefulness. The technology adoption questionnaire probed three categories of usefulness – perceived usefulness, perceived trust, and satisfaction with the eWhiteboard. Table 20 summarizes the responses. There was no doubt as to the perceived benefits - all respondents rated them highly. In an open question, the respondents listed two major reasons for the high ratings - reduced phone calls (related to patient status and patient transfer) and "knowing" the current patient status. As for the disadvantages, respondents seemed to vary their ratings from one extreme to the other – the main disadvantage they listed in the open question was that during their busy days "one may forget to update the status or may update the wrong field".

On the issue of perceived trust, clinicians reported being "upset" and "curious" when they receive phone calls for patients under their care that have a correctly indicated status on the eWhiteboard. Most respondents attributed such unwarranted calls to their colleagues' "lack of confidence in the whiteboard" and lack of proficiency in using it ("they don't know how to use the whiteboard"). When the status for a patient under their team's care was not correctly updated on the eWhiteboard, the majority of respondents were "curious how it happened". (Table 10 and Table 20 refer to the same types of *trust* situations – Table 10 shows observed behaviors, while Table 20 reflects perceptions)

The overall satisfaction with the introduction of the eWhiteboard into the work process of the surgical system was rated very high.

Table 20. Questionnaire responses.

	Question	Rating (Likert scale)		Reasons (% represents how many people listed the reason as one of their answers)	
perceived usefulness	advantages	1 (no advantage)	0%	less calls	80%
		2	0%	knowing patient status	30%
		3	0%	not specified	10%
		4	50%		
		5 (improves my work)	50%		
	disadvantages	1 (no disadvantage)	40%	"one may forget to update status or may update the wrong field"	30%
		2	20%		
		3	20%	"we still get calls for patients"	20%
		4	10%	"people don't know how to use the whiteboard"	10%
		5 (many disadvantages)	10%	"we need more information displayed"	10%
				"implementation is not through the continuum of care"	10%
				"no disadvantages"	10%
				not specified	20%
trust	How do you feel when you get a call for a patient whose status on the whiteboard is accurate?			upset	40%
				curious	40%
				doesn't bother me	10%
				angry	10%
	Why do you think you get such calls?			They don't trust my work, they're checking on me	20%
				They don't know how to use the whiteboard	70%
				They are making sure everything is ok	30%
				Lack of confidence in the whiteboard	80%
	How do you feel when you get a call for a patient whose status on the whiteboard is INACCURATE?			guilty	20%
				upset	0%
				curious how it happened	60%
				doesn't bother me	20%
satisfaction	How satisfied are you with the introduction of the whiteboard as a communication tool?				
		1 (not at all)	0%		
		2	0%		
		3	10%		
		4	40%		
		5 (very much)	50%		

4.5 Discussion of findings

This research employed the activity theory and workflow analysis perspectives in the study of breakdowns in surgical care coordination with a systems engineering approach. Through the examination of people, processes, artifacts and procedures in-situ, several important socio-organizational factors were identified as barriers to efficient and safe coordination of patient care. These factors included conflicting interests and mistrust between micro-systems, the challenge of system-wide situation awareness, as well as the constraints of physical spaces. These qualitative findings regarding the work practice provided meaningful background and explanation for the quantitative component of the research. The following discussion presents the integration of both.

A relatively low number of breakdowns were observed over a long period of time demonstrating an overall reliable and smooth process. This is consistent with findings from other clinical settings [121]. Contrary to expectations, no issues with implicit intra-team coordination were found. Reliance on spatial and visual cues as signifiers of activity status was prominent – e.g. placement of objects, highlights and notes, but no significant efforts or breakdowns were associated with this type of collaborative work. This can be explained by the fact that implicit coordination was utilized by means of procedural conventions in routine tasks, rather than in novel or out of the ordinary situations. Thus, in this study, implicit coordination was not found to be problematic in relation to safety, but rather facilitated an economic way of coordination in routine patient care work.

Significant effort and a number of breakdowns were observed with inter-team coordination that was explicit. A similar observation was reported by [243]. Unlike the instances of implicit coordination, the explicit coordination episodes concerned non-scripted coordination tasks. In fact, most often inter-team explicit coordination breakdowns centered around novel or unexpected situations. One major issue in these cases was maintenance of system-wide situation awareness among all teams. Another problem was reaching agreement on action plans when teams' interests collided. Previous research in an OR suite has also indicated that the need to reconcile multiple conflicting goals is a complicating factor to perioperative work that leads to opportunities for error and to compromises in patient safety [246]. The results suggest that the best target for process or technological support is at micro-system boundaries (i.e. inter-team) in the continuum of the socio-technical care macro-system, and in decision support for inter-professional coordination. The main information needs of clinicians through the surgical process – patient care, patient status, OR schedule status, and OR status – can provide a good starting point for technology to address those problematic inter-team coordination efforts.

This study confirmed the reports by Ren et al. that breakdowns originate throughout the surgical system and at any time [243]. An important novel finding of this research is that inter-team coordination breakdowns often propagate downstream in the surgical system process, which effects increased communication cost associated with repair. This is due to the fact that as they propagate, breakdowns affect the work of a greater number of people, as well as due to the increased criticality of process inputs as a patient approaches surgery. To minimize risk and reduce process waste, the opportunities for breakdown propagation need to be diminished. The implication is that stricter measures are necessary so that all inputs at transition points in patient care are in place. Instead of breakdowns being disablers of patient care, disablers of breakdowns should be embedded in the process. These ideas are further developed in Chapter 6.

This research found several dependencies between tangibility and other breakdown properties. For example, the tangibility of the coordination process relates to the breakdown theme. This finding indicates that particular types of information need (*i.e.* the breakdown theme) are communicated through specific coordination mechanisms (*i.e.* the tangibility). The tangibility did not exhibit a correlation to coordination scale. Thus, the type of coordination mechanism employed does not bear influence on whether a breakdown will affect one team or multiple teams. In other words, tangible and intangible coordination mechanisms are equally relevant to breakdowns that affect intra- and inter-team work. Further, the tangibility of the coordination process was found to correlate with the repair strategy employed. This means that the coordination mechanism related to a breakdown determines the type of repair mechanism that will be utilized to fix the breakdown.

The findings also revealed several insights related to the breakdown repair strategy employed. In Hospital_1, it was found that the breakdown type correlates with the repair strategy. This was not the case in Hospital_2. A likely explanation for this difference is the distribution of breakdowns by type in the data for Hospital_2. Human error and technical breakdowns were observed very few times in Hospital_2 (see Table 10). This could explain the lack of association found between breakdown type and repair strategy. The research also showed that the breakdown theme correlates with the repair strategy, in both hospitals. Thus, the particular type of information need related to the breakdown (*i.e.* the breakdown theme) is associated with a specific type of repair mechanism employed in the breakdown resolution.

Another critical finding of this work is the role of breakdowns in inducing interruptions to clinicians' work. A significant body of research has demonstrated the contributing effects of interruptions to adverse events and medical error in healthcare work [62, 81, 97]. In this study, interruptions comprise a subset of the possible communication chunks that make up the full set of chunk types defining a breakdown repair cost[4]. Therefore, while it is not surprising that there is a strong relationship between interruptions and breakdowns communication cost, the significance lies in the fact that the relationship can be quantified. Further, that a predictive power can be established. This study determined that breakdowns in routine patient care, specifically the communication overhead associated with their repair, are a major source of interruptions. In addition, this study revealed that despite the high degree of similarity in the occurrence of breakdowns in the two hospitals, the impact of breakdowns can vary from one organization to another, depending on such factors as the culture of communication – whether it is one of proactive pre-emptive information diffusion that effects the development of formalized communication patterns, or one of reactive information distribution that relies on information pull when an information need arises.

The results highlight the need to examine issues of large scale coordination in detail in order to derive recommendations for operational optimization and technological support that will minimize breakdown lifetime and consequently repair costs and interruptions. In turn, this focus will improve efficiency and reduce the potential for safety risks. In the following, the findings are abstracted and placed within an initial theoretical framework positioned in the context of theories of coordination in organizations. Then a model of safety outcomes during breakdown situations is offered. Lastly, the role of *trust* in technology adoption is discussed.

4.5.1 Conceptual model of breakdowns in the surgical process

Several models of coordination and cooperation in response to breakdowns have been proposed within organizational sciences. In this section, the findings of this study are positioned at the crossroads of two such frameworks by combining and extending their assumptions to produce a model of coordination work and breakdowns for the OR work setting.

The framework of [181] situates group coordination within a pattern of relationships among task structure, organizational structure, awareness and communication. The essential postulate of the model is that the organizational structure interacts with the nature of the tasks at hand to produce and affect the need for coordination among team members, which in turn produces and affects the need for communication (Figure 21). The particular instance of all these variables determines team performance.

---

[4] Chunk types that are not interruptions include writing a note, filling in a request form, interacting with the electronic systems

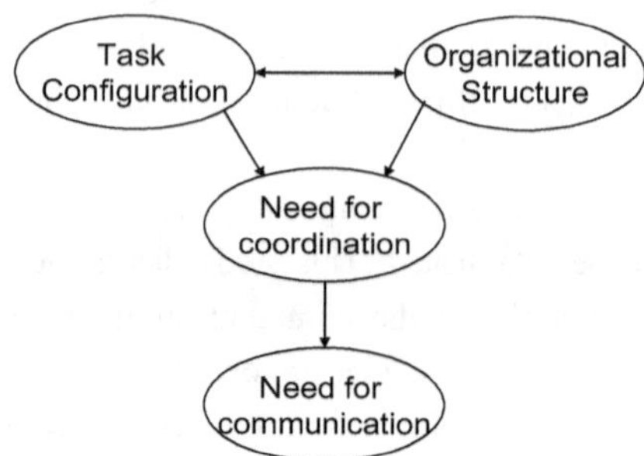

Figure 21: Model of coordination, abbreviated - from [181].

The model of cooperation by [291] was developed with a larger unit of analysis in terms of scale of coordination - it comes from the context of inter-organizational cooperation. This model reflects the processes of coordination that are employed as a response to unexpected events. The premise is that disturbances and unexpected events result in collective process-related actions that aim to bring the state of the socio-technical system to the initial state of coordinatedness. Depending on the degree of cooperation required to accomplish a stable coordination state, the model defines that either *corrective cooperation* (e.g. workarounds) will occur, or *remediative coordination* (if larger scale solutions are necessary such as persistent organizational solutions). The detailed model description is presented in Figure 22.

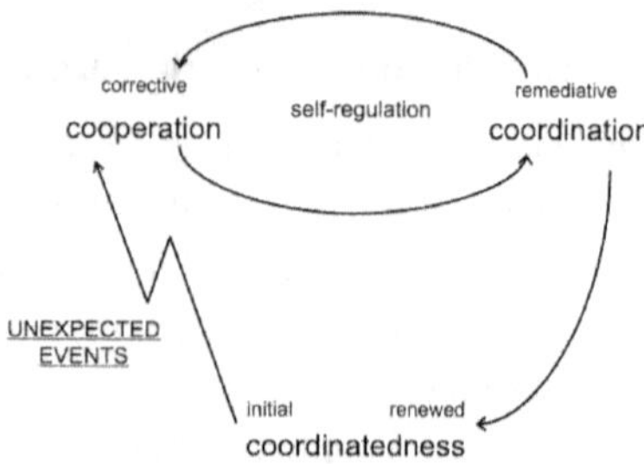

Figure 22: Model of cooperation, abbreviated - from [291].

Combining some of the constructs from the two models described above with the findings of this work, a conceptual framework of coordination and breakdowns in OR operations is derived (Figure 23). As in the first model presented above, the *Organizational Structure* interacts with the *Task Configuration*, and together they effect the *Need for Coordination*. The

Coordination Theme and the *Tangibility of Coordination* are closely-coupled parameters of coordination – *i.e.* influencing each other – that determine the specific *Need for Communication.* The Organizational Structure defines the formal coordination tools and options for flexible rules, standards and conventions, and therefore influences the Tangibility of Coordination in a given situation. Task Configuration is related to the Coordination Theme. The Task Configuration, Organizational Structure, Coordination Theme, Tangibility of Coordination, and communication are the mechanisms that bond the disparate activities of surgical teams into a coherent flow that makes the surgical patient care. It is referred to as a *Normal State* of the perioperative system.

The Need for Communication among agents in the activity is not always successfully realized, or unexpected events happen, in which case a *Breakdown* occurs (The construct of breakdown reflects the notion of unexpected events and disturbances from Wehner et al.'s framework [291]. Thus, the rest of the discussion of unexpected events and disturbances is framed by referring to these as breakdowns). The OR system state changes to *Breakdown State* which poses a *Need for Re-coordination* through repair work in order to bring the surgical system back to normal operation. The Coordination Theme implicitly defines the breakdown theme at the moment when a breakdown occurs. Repair efforts are initiated upon breakdown detection.

The Need for Re-coordination demands that agents choose and adopt a *Repair Strategy.* The choice of Repair Strategy is related to the Coordination Theme and the Tangibility of the broken process of coordination. Repair Strategy determines the specific *Need for Communication,* which in turn initiates the actual *Repair Work.* The notion of *Repair Work* is inclusive of the concepts of corrective cooperation and remediative coordination from [291]'s model.

The Organizational Structure determines the range of possible breakdown propagation. Hence, *Breakdown Lifetime* is dependent on the Organizational Structure. The *Repair Cost* is determined by the Breakdown Lifetime. Upon successful repair, the system resumes its *Normal State.*

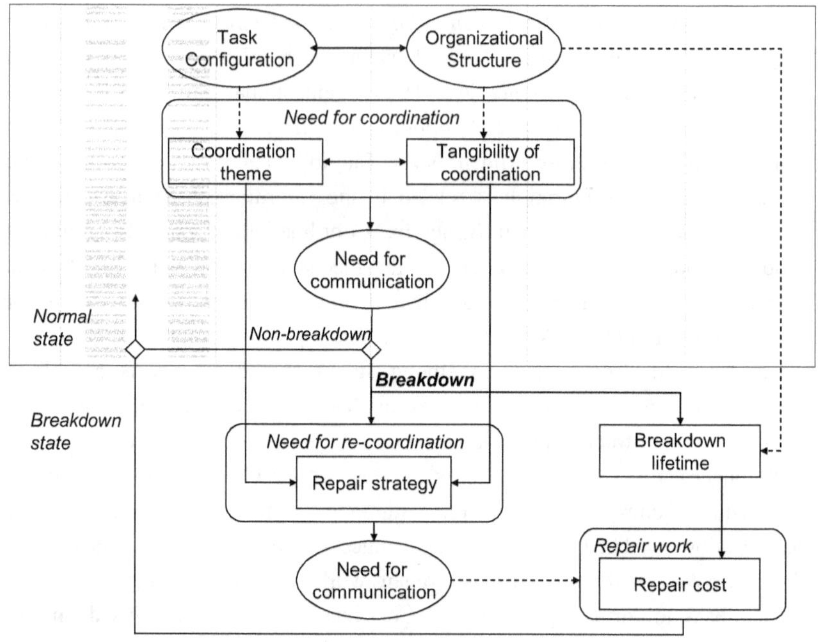

Figure 23: Abstract representation of the factors influencing breakdowns and repairs in the perioperative system. Solid arrows represent relationships established by this work and by that of [181]. Dotted arrows indicate links derived by theory.

The suggested framework provides a diagrammatical reflection of the relationships among variables that were found in this study. Through this study an appreciation of the deeper features of breakdowns is achieved from a process-oriented perspective. The conceptual model facilitates an improved understanding of the dependencies of organizational mechanisms and their relationship to breakdowns.

4.5.2 Conceptual model of safety and breakdowns

Good coordination does not affect performance until workload is extremely high [112]. Assuming that high communication cost is inherently an indicator of heightened workload (as the communication itself is an additional load to existing taskload), it is this notion – that the outcome of a high workload, high stress, high uncertainty situation is a function of the 'goodness' of coordination – that can shed light to the one very significant difference found between Hospital_1 and

Hospital_2. Despite the great number of similarities between the two hospitals, one important difference was found – unlike Hospital_1, the highest-cost breakdowns at Hospital_2 presented a safety risk. This can be explained through the lens of the qualitative findings. At Hospital_1, more strictly defined roles and communication channels resulted in the creation of formal conventions for the re-coordination of activity among multiple micro-systems upon breakdowns – *i.e.* the coordination patterns (see Section 4.2.3). The communication culture of Hospital_1 can be defined as one of proactive pre-emptive information diffusion. The utilization of coordination patterns presented a small communication overhead in return for minimizing the risk of inducing further breakdowns and compromising safety. The process structure at Hospital_2 was designed to allow for greater flexibility and a lower level of formalism. As a result, while there existed common ground (i.e. shared understanding) of what a breakdown resolution should entail, breakdown repairs did not follow a strict script of actions but rather were resolved on an ad hoc basis. The culture of communication was reactive in nature – information was sought and distributed when needed, rather than broadcast to the attention of all micro-systems. Consequently, the greater level of uncertainty at Hospital_2 (due to the bigger unit size and the association with a trauma centre) in combination with the lack of formalized communication channels for breakdown resolution led to conditions in which breakdown repair work often triggered the emergence of new breakdowns and impacted safety.

Based on the above insights, the conceptual model of safety in Figure 24 was developed. The model proposes that several parameters affect the occurrence of *breakdowns*. The *communication culture, stakeholders' interests* that can collide at any one moment in time, the *process structure* (e.g. flexible and distributed or hierarchical with functional allocations) *and* the *amount of dynamic conditions* affecting clinical coordination are the critical parameters that surfaced as a result of this study. The list of parameters can certainly be expanded with further research.

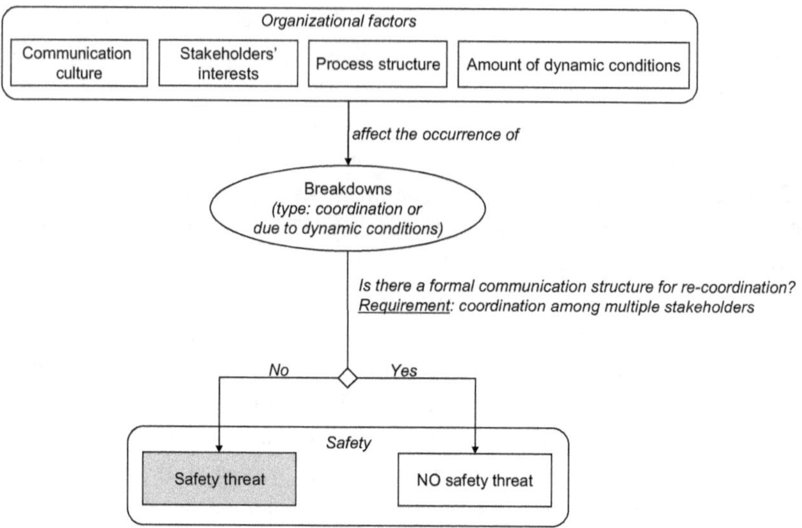

Figure 24: Model of safety for surgical unit operations.

The data of this study revealed that high-cost breakdowns are of the type *coordination* and *coordination due to dynamic conditions*. Upon the instantiation of a *Breakdown* situation, the requirement for repair from the breakdown is that coordination must be negotiated with multiple stakeholders/micro-systems. The crucial factor in the outcome of the breakdown – whether it will potentially threaten patient safety, is the presence of established *formal communication structure for re-coordination*. Such structures were present in the case of Hospital_1 information broadcast protocols. It is assumed, however, that any formalized communication tool can be utilized including computer-mediated communication solutions.

The model helps to understand the relationship between several organizational factors, breakdowns and safety. It can be concluded that a more 'proactive' approach to handling re-coordination upon breakdowns, such as establishing protocols of communication, is more effective at minimizing safety risks than a 'reactive' approach that deals with issues of coordination at the spur of the moment. Such understanding can facilitate the informed design of breakdown disablers and communication tools that target improved safety and efficiency.

4.5.3 The role of trust in adoption

The role of trust - a socio-organizational culture factor, was found to be a key factor for successful adoption of communication technology such as the eWhiteboard. The eWhiteboard achieved the goal of reducing communication load among care providers. Further, it significantly reduced coordination breakdowns related to awareness of the status of things. However, the findings confirmed that success of implementation is defined in the eyes of the beholder. While overall communication load and awareness breakdowns were reduced, and perceptions of usefulness and satisfaction were very positive, the qualitative and quantitative metrics of communication overhead revealed several negative outcomes.

First, the observations in Phase 2 unequivocally showed that patient status coordination was not completely achieved via the eWhiteboard, but was still partially mediated over the phone. Qualitative analysis of participants' comments led to the conclusion that the persisting phone calls were triggered by a deep systemic issue – lack of trust in the work of other humans. Specifically, the lack of trust was exhibited at inter-team boundaries – *i.e.* between micro-systems, which is the dimension that the eWhiteboard was supposed to facilitate communication over. The following situation was observed numerous times: a participant using the eWhiteboard chose to confirm or question the information via the phone despite observing a clear patient status on the eWhiteboard display. This behavior meant that the respective party questioned whether "*they*" updated the patient status. The observations indicated that most of the time the eWhiteboard was accurately updated. There were, however, a few cases when the information was not current.

During the study at Hospital_2, evidence for lack of trust in the work of other teams was observed as well, even though it was unrelated to technology implementation. For instance, a nurse in one of the patient care areas checked the test results for a patient in the electronic system, saying "I'd like to check and make sure they are not abnormal because I am afraid somebody in OR won't check". Also, nurses and coordinators were seen always double-checking the information provided to them by physicians regarding bed availability in the hospital, because they suspected that physicians compete with each other for providing beds for their patients and therefore provide inaccurate information. Similar to Hospital_1, dissatisfaction and frustration with inter-team coordination was also expressed: "they are in this department because they're supposed to use their heads". These examples from Hospital_2, although informally reported here, support the findings from Hospital_1 that reveal the critical impact that the organizational culture and specifically the attitude towards the work of other teams has on communication workload and consequently on breakdowns and adoption.

Similar to the success stories reported in many accounts of clinical implementations, the self-reported perception measures in the study of technology adoption at Hospital_1 indicate well received technology adoption and high satisfaction. This is not surprising given the main objective of reducing communication load was achieved. What is surprising are the questionnaire responses on the issue of *trust* (Table 20). The communication overhead was perceived by all but one person as lack of trust in the actual eWhiteboard and lack of proficiency on others' part in using the technology. The observations, however, showed that the use-errors associated with the eWhiteboard were not relevant to the few situations when a care provider failed to execute an update and therefore the information on a patient was not current. Instead, use-errors were associated with slips during updates. For example, during execution of an update of patient status, the nurse unintentionally selects several patient rows on the eWhiteboard, which results in changing the status for all of them. Use errors were immediately corrected – the nurse always noticed the erroneous update and re-updated the eWhiteboard. The observations did not indicate lack of proficiency with using the tool – therefore it is concluded that the lack of trust in other people is possibly projected onto the eWhiteboard, which mediates the communication between 'us' and 'them'.

Having quantified the observational data allowed to achieve a description of the unanticipated issues in technology adoption that spans beyond a qualitative narrative. It was found that along with reduction in patient care communication, the eWhiteboard's utilization was accompanied by a significant overhead that is unaccounted for in survey metrics. The issue of trust comprised a major portion of coordination breakdowns recorded in Phase 2, and therefore to a great extent it demotes the success of the eWhiteboard. In this sense, the findings confirm the double-sided adoption accounts reported by others.

It is worth noting that in the case of healthcare, communication of accurate and timely information is critical. In this sense, lack of trust as exhibited in persistent phone calls to confirm and question information is not necessarily a negative behavior. The lack of trust could be seen as the efforts that collaborators invest in ensuring reliability of the larger socio-technical system. The environment is complex and hectic. Maintaining safe patient care operations, as well as optimizing efficiency in order to avoid losing revenue (as in the following example), are the drivers of such behaviors. Oftentimes, critical decisions regarding changes in the plan of care need to be made based on real-time status information that may not be reflected on a manual update status display for several minutes – *e.g.* "has the patient arrived in the hospital in this precise moment of time or should we start preparing another patient for the same OR". The consequence, as seen in this study, is communication overhead. Hence, future system designs should aim to ensure the maintenance of reliable operations with real-time information, in a way that ameliorates potential inter-team/micro-system mistrust.

4.6 Chapter summary

Between the two hospitals studied, a great number of commonalities were found: similar safety culture, information needs of clinicians, equivalent number and types of breakdowns that occur, and comparable communication overhead. What became clear in both hospital contexts was that breakdowns stem from failing coordination between different teams in patient care, *i.e.* between micro-system interfaces. When a breakdown occurred, it often propagated downstream in the surgical care process. Properties of the breakdown determined properties of repair. The distance a breakdown propagated before detection and repair positively correlated with the communication cost that fixing the breakdown incurred. The breakdown repair cost was also a major source of interruptions to clinical work.

Although largely similar in breakdown behavior, the two surgical units differed in one dimension – the safety risk potential of their most difficult to resolve breakdowns. Analysis led to the conclusion that safety is at least partially dependent on the availability of pre-established communication protocols for dealing with breakdowns.

The study of adoption revealed that trust in other humans is a complex issue that underlies partial resistance to completely embracing the benefits of communication technology.

In the next chapters the insights from a better understanding of the anatomy of breakdowns will be developed into a method for breakdown detection and a framework for the management of breakdowns.

5
Breakdown Detection

This chapter develops a breakdown detection method as a useful approach to the management of breakdowns in inter-team coordination within the context of the daily operations of surgical units. The method is based on breakdown detection approaches in other domains and on insights acquired through this study. The chapter begins with a survey of the theoretical background for the method, shows its utility through a sample analysis, and concludes with a presentation of the validation of the method. Limitations are discussed as well.

The costly overhead of re-coordination effort following a breakdown, along with the safety risks introduced to clinical work by means of interruptions and cognitive overload, require that breakdowns be managed so that perioperative coordination is achieved in an economic and safe fashion. The finding of this and other research indicate that systemic level factors represent the main contributors to everyday breakdowns. These findings point to the significance of inter-operability at the micro-system interface (e.g. inter-professional or inter-team communication), as well as the technical interface of new implementations. With the current worldwide move to digitize all healthcare information, the need to integrate information within a socio-technical system such as a hospital is especially pertinent. However, this is not a trivial task. The literature abounds with examples of partially successful implementations that result in resistance to adoption, increased patient safety concerns, increased breakdowns, and changed workflows in unanticipated ways [160, 319].

The first step towards the management of breakdowns is the ability to detect them. To address the issues of technology implementation at the micro-system interface, as well as to reduce safety threats arising from breakdowns, there is a need for a better assessment of the presence of breakdowns at the macro system level in healthcare processes. This chapter will present a method for breakdown detection that provides a systematic approach to both manual and automatic inter-team (*i.e.* macro-system level) breakdown detection. The goal of the method is to identify the amount of pre- and post-implementation, or pre- and post-intervention, breakdowns in perioperative work. This can be accomplished either in real-time or retrospectively (based on communication records). The method aims to provide a practical way of detecting breakdowns that occur between different teams – at large-scale coordination, based on criteria derived from empirical findings. The management of breakdowns will be discussed in Chapter 6.

5.1 Target detection points

The great majority of breakdowns in coordination were found relevant to inter-team processes. In half of the cases, those same breakdowns affected intra-team work as well. Very few breakdowns were related to coordination at the intra-team dimension only. Therefore, the detection method described in this chapter is focused on the discovery of inter-team breakdowns.

The detection of breakdowns is possible at the point when a repair occurs and therefore has a post hoc monitoring nature – breakdowns are not prevented from happening but are identified upon repair. This approach is suitable for the detection of breakdowns in the surgical process as the occurrence of a breakdown is unknown until detection, at which time a repair action is initiated.

5.2 Breakdown detection approaches

Breakdown detection is characterized by a suspicion that an error/breakdown has occurred, independent from understanding the nature and causes behind it [316]. Despite the need to better understand and utilize breakdown detection mechanisms in order to improve safety, while recognizing that not all breakdowns can be prevented, research on error management in the safety-critical domains such as aviation has focused primarily on the development of error classification schemes, the design of error tolerant systems, and error prevention through training and design [250]. Very few studies investigate the problem of breakdown detection in high-risk domains [250].

Consequently, only several approaches to breakdown detection in aviation have been offered thus far. Some focus on the cognitive aspects of breakdown detection, narrowing in on the human as the grain of analysis [158, 250] – examining the potential for people in the socio-technical system to apply strategies for breakdown detection. Cognitive approaches, however, are not easily translated to the macro-system process framework where inter-team coordination is the focal point. Another approach in aviation exploits computational linguistics analysis methods in the examination of communication patterns and their relation to error and performance in the cockpit – the overall number of words spoken, the length of words, and other linguistic dimensions in the communication of crew members [259].

A third methodology examines communication patterns analysis in air traffic control, albeit not specifically breakdown detection, and draws the attention to the flow of information [37]. Yet another approach converges solely on the monitoring of activity based on a predefined model of expected behavior and detects breakdowns by identifying deviations in actual behavior [46]. This latter construct of comparing prescribed and actual behavior is in fact common to all breakdown and error detection methods [283]. Given that breakdown detection research and practice in aviation, and in safety-critical domains in general, has yet to mature, the following review looks at non-risk domains that offer a solid scientific and practical background in breakdown detection approaches. It is these approaches that have inspired the aforementioned work in aviation.

The detection of breakdowns has been extensively studied in a variety of disciplines such as conversation analysis, second language acquisition, speech pathology and computational linguistics. Although these disciplines are concerned with the study of breakdowns at the conversational level as opposed to the larger scale inter-team coordination level, both levels of analysis share an important commonality - the underlying mechanism of interest behind conversation and large-scale coordination is communication. Thus, insights acquired in the context of conversation can be used as a foundational framework for the development of the large-scale coordination breakdowns detection method. The following will focus on the review of the major approaches from the field of computational linguistics for several reasons. First, computational linguistics offers several decades of sound scientific research on the topic of breakdown detection. Second, computational linguistics methods are inspired by the other disciplines' wisdom and therefore represent a unified body of knowledge. Third, the breakdown detection methods are not concerned with language processing per se. The methods focus on the dynamics and structure of communication – an approach that easily translates beyond the original domain.

In the context of speech, breakdown detection is understood to be the monitoring of dialog for cues that some miscommunication (*i.e.* breakdown) has occurred [193]. The recognition of breakdowns, *i.e.* the identification of cues, is accomplished through computational models of interactional structures. There are two approaches to the modeling of interaction – grammar-based and plan-based [260]. Grammar-based models embody knowledge about the linguistic structure of dialog. Plan-based models infer mental states of agents via sets of rules that aid the inference of task-related plans – that is, plan-based models incorporate knowledge about the structure of the task at hand. More sophisticated models combine both approaches [192]. The interactional models are used to generate predictions about user behaviors. Each deviation of user behavior from dialog predictions is interpreted as a signal of the potential occurrence of breakdowns [69].

Predictions allow a system to detect breakdowns in communication in two ways. On the one hand, expectations about the content of the next interactional contribution allow the system to accept or reject an interpretation of user's conversational contribution. For example, an automated travel agent system can have the following set of predictions about the task of selling a travel ticket [69]:

1. A statement about the name of the departure city
2. A statement about the name of the departure city and other required parameters, such as the date and the time of departure
3. An explicit confirmation of the arrival, and the departure city
4. An explicit denial of the understood arrival city and a request for another arrival city
5. An explicit denial of the understood arrival city

Based on the set of predictions, the system can accept a limited number of speech acts and reject others that don't comply with the expectations. However, even the accepted interactions may constitute a breakdown. For example, name confusion of the departure city – the user says "Roma" and the system interprets it as "Arona". In such a case, the breakdown will propagate through the interaction contributed by the system, and will be consequently detected by the user who is better able to identify the breakdown. At this point, the user will adopt a repair strategy, which will represent a deviation from the next predicted behavior. This deviation presents the second way in which the system detects breakdowns – by noting the empirical consequence in the user's response. A different type of expectation related to the interpretation of user behavior will trigger repair efforts by the system. For example [69]:

6. A statement including a new arrival city, plus the departure city
7. A statement including a new arrival city

Without an explicit negation statement by the user, through predictions (6) and (7) the system can still determine that the new statements represent an implicit negation and an initiation of repair – the user asks the system to return to the context where miscommunication occurred. Predictions of this type, where implicit meaning is interpreted, are derived by research across disciplines – conversation analysis, linguistics, second language acquisition, and speech pathology.

The breakdown detection approaches described above are the backbone of a variety of computational models. Each model extends the detection capability in a certain direction. One model incorporates conversational context analysis in the interpretation of breakdowns [69]. Another combines plan-based predictions with expectations derived from social norms [192]. Other approaches utilize Bayesian networks to identify the source of breakdowns and maximize mutual understanding [218].

In summary, breakdown detection in computational linguistics does not involve language processing, but is achieved through modeling of interactional structure – either linguistic structure or task structure. Based on the models, a set of formal expectations is derived, which can include context-independent rules, domain specific predictions and expectations derived from social norms. These predictions are exploited as constraints on user behavior. When a non-expected action is observed at the conversation level, the system reasons a breakdown has occurred. Table 21 summarizes the computational linguistics approach.

Table 21. Requirements for a method of breakdown detection

Requirements for breakdown detection
1. Model a structure of interaction
2. Derive predictions from the structural model
3. Detect breakdowns based on predictions

5.3 Method of detection

This section develops a detection analysis framework that facilitates inter-team breakdown detection for the surgical setting. The method is based on the breakdown detection models from the field of computational linguistics, where interactional structure is modeled and determines interactional predictions, which implicitly define the occurrence of breakdowns. The computational linguistics models concern the coordination of conversation between a system and a user. Thus, application of the breakdown detection approach to large-scale coordination, such as surgical inter-team coordination, must extend the scope of analysis to accommodate the domain requirements by preserving the core approach while incorporating knowledge about coordination acquired through this and previous studies of perioperative work.

Detecting breakdowns of inter-team coordination scale requires the analysis of communication between teams rather than between a single user and a single system. In the inter-team context, information is exchanged among more than two interactional objects (i.e. teams/micro-systems), and therefore can be characterized by a *flow* – a notion that reflects the trajectory a particular information instance travels in terms of its communication to and from different micro-systems in the surgical system. Coordination between teams revolves around the exchange of different types of domain-specific information by means of communication. Therefore, each type of information will follow a particular flow within the surgical process. The common goal among teams is to provide efficient and safe patient care, while each team is carrying out independent but concurrent tasks that need to be coordinated by means of information exchange. Hence, while breakdowns between a user and a system are detected through an examination of the bi-directional communication of information between them, the focus of analysis for the inter-team coordination context is the *information flow* for the various types of domain-relevant information exchanged between any two teams.

The information flow provides the equivalent of an interactional structure model, as information flow is commonly formally defined within each organization and unit. Thus, a mapping of the information flow can be obtained without the high cost of analysis. For finer-grained breakdown detection or in the case that information flow mapping is not readily available, interviewing clinicians at each process step can solicit the required flow information. Information flow provides a reflection of the domain-specific task structure, with a main focus on communication of information at the macro-system process level.

Following the identification of the different types of information and their trajectories, predictions of communication behavior defining a *normal state* of the system can be derived. Depending on the scope of analysis required, predictions can be extrapolated from additional sources such as empirical research. The prediction inference options are:

1. Generate predictions about information flow based on existing information flow mapping. These predictions should be per type of domain-specific information (e.g. patient chart, consent, lab tests, emergency cases, bed availability), and can be uni- or bi-directional relationships of communication between micro-systems.
2. Generate/refine predictions about information flow as related to the properties of coordination (e.g. tangibility of coordination, theme, etc.). Such predictions are derived based on this and other studies, as well as on local empirical data. The predictions can be uni- or bi-directional relationships of communication between micro-systems.[5]
   - If a relationship between properties exists, communication predictions should be generated with constraints – *i.e.* a cross-check that the expected relationship is maintained. For example, in the present study it was established that a breakdown's theme relates to the tangibility of the coordination process. Thus, if a patient status inquiry is executed over an expectation for intangible coordination – an indication of a breakdown will be triggered[5]. Conceptual model representations such as the one described in Section 4.5.1 can be particularly helpful in correctly establishing all constraints.
3. Generate predictions about information flow and properties of coordination derived from social norms at the surgical unit of coordination. This step requires actual empirical research investment. The benefit is the inclusion of important criteria such as organizational culture factors – *i.e.* conventions of communication, and patterns of coordination (as in Chapter 4, Section 4.2.3). These can produce *normal state* predictions, or *breakdown state* expectations – the determination requires knowledge of the work practice. Constraints linking a potential breakdown to safety can be established, such

[5] In the current study, the identified properties' relationships pertain to breakdowns and would therefore establish predictions of the presence of breakdowns. However, 'normal' state predictions based on relationships among properties can be established based on other studies.

as those discussed in Chapter 4, Section 4.5.2.

Based on the predictions set forth in 1-3 above, a potential breakdown is detected when a communication instance does not satisfy any of the information flow predictions, and/or it adheres to one of the breakdown expectations. Detection occurs at the point of breakdown repair as the communication instance at repair would violate a prediction. In other words, information would be sought from a team that should have provided it and thus the flow will go in the opposite direction of the expected prediction. Communications that go against the direction of prediction between any two teams are a deviation and can be inferred a potential breakdown. Detection occurs at the repair point as well in the case of communication behavior that matches a breakdown expectation.

Optionally, the detection method can be improved with higher degree of detection validity. At the moment of detection the first repair strategy is detected as well. One of the constraints identified through this work is that the repair strategy is determined by the tangibility and theme of coordination. Therefore, further intelligence to the detection method can be implemented by adding a check that verifies the detected repair strategy matches the expected repair strategy (thus, a set of predictions of repair strategies must be implemented). The outcome of this verification process determines the strength of probability that the detected breakdown is in fact a breakdown.

Finally, a history of valid breakdown detections can be stored over time and used as part of the breakdown detection validation phase. If the detected event matches a 'context' stored in the history, then the strength of probability of a valid breakdown detection is increased.

The method is summarized in Table 22.

Table 22. Breakdown detection method

Requirements	Method
1. Model a structure of interaction	*Model the information flow at the process level for the different types of domain-relevant information*
2. Derive predictions from the structural model	*Determine direction of information flow between all teams for the following predictions:* *a) Generate predictions based on existing information flow mapping. These are per type of domain-specific information (e.g. patient chart, consent, lab tests, emergency cases, bed availability)* *b) Generate/refine predictions related to the properties of coordination (e.g. tangibility, theme). Predictions are derived from research. Implement cross-checks to ensure cross-property constraints are maintained, if necessary.* *c) Generate predictions of breakdown behavior* *d) Generate predictions derived from social norms* *e) (optional) Generate predictions for repair strategies based on research* *f) (optional) Store a history of valid breakdown detections*
3. Detect breakdowns based on predictions	*- Communications that go against the direction of prediction between any two teams are a deviation and can be inferred a potential breakdown* *- Communications that conform to breakdown expectations are inferred a potential breakdown* *- (optional) Validate the potential breakdown by comparing actual repair with expected repair* *- (optional) Validate the potential breakdown by comparing to the history data*

5.4 Validation

Validation of the breakdown detection method is crucial in establishing the usefulness of the method in providing meaningful outcomes. The diagnostic performance of algorithms is commonly evaluated with analysis of the Receiver Operating Characteristic (ROC) curve. This analysis method has been extensively applied in a variety of domains such as medical and biomedical informatics [166, 296], clinical decision-making and clinical medicine [78, 195, 227, 320], social sciences [267, 268], machine learning [96, 165, 262], and others. ROC curve analysis examines the true positive and false positive rates produced at each detection level. This allows the analyst to determine whether the diagnostic test's output reflects a reasonable rate of valid detection or approximates a random detection rate.

The breakdown detection method is a binary classification algorithm – it classifies events as either being a breakdown or not. Breakdown events that are detected are referred to as true positives (TP), whereas those that are not detected are false negatives (FN). Events that are not breakdowns and do not trigger detection are known as true negatives (TN). Non-breakdown events that trigger a detection are referred to as false positives (FP). The false positive rate (FPR) measures the percentage of non-breakdown events that have triggered the method to return a detection and have therefore been misclassified. The true positive rate (TPR) measures the percentage of correctly classified breakdowns as compared to all the breakdowns in the test sample.

ROC curve analysis plots the TPR against the FPR as the detection sensitivity is varied. The analysis is commonly used to evaluate discrete classifiers, including binary classifiers – tests that classify objects on the basis of the existence of some property. As such, ROC curve analysis is the most appropriate validation tool for the breakdown detection method.

The applicability and accuracy of the breakdown detection method can be evaluated by measuring its performance at variable levels of breakdown detection sensitivity. A basic set of communication flow predictions was derived for Hospital_1 and Hospital_2. The level of breakdown detection was adjusted by reducing the number of initial predictions. The following sections elaborate on the procedures. ROC analysis of the resulting performance of the breakdown detection method revealed excellent performance over the data for both hospitals.

5.4.1 Structure of interaction – information flow

The information flows for each type of domain-specific coordinative information were defined for Hospital_1 – phases 1 and 2, and for Hospital_2, based on workflow knowledge acquired in the early stages of this study through interviewing and observations (see Chapter 3) in combination with information flow diagrams provided by the perioperative unit management. The aim of validation was to evaluate the method with a most basic set of predictions and therefore the focus of information flow analysis examined only the outgoing and incoming phone calls for each team in the surgical process. An additional factor considered was the use of the electronic patient record system that was known to indicate that some *patient information* was missing in the patient chart.

The information flow model for each hospital represents an ideally coordinated process for that hospital – *i.e.* the goal information flow for all types of information. The major domain-specific information types that comprised the models are equivalent to the information foci and themes identified in this study – *e.g.* patient status, OR readiness, schedule, etc.

Figure 25 shows the information flow model expected for ideally coordinated breakdown-free communication among teams on the day of surgery for Hospital_1, Phase 1. Any type of phone communication between teams that is not reflected in the model, including phone calls to teams that are not represented in the figure (e.g. communication to/from the Booking team, Surgeon's office, external services, etc.), is considered a potential breakdown. The information flows for Hospital_1, Phase 2, and for Hospital_2 were analogously modeled and can be found in the Appendix C.1.

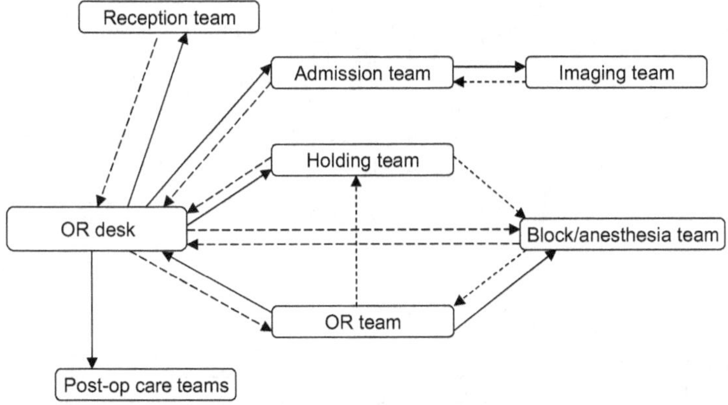

Figure 25: Day of surgery information flow model for Hospital_1, Phase_1. Solid arrows represent allowable phone communication between teams on any type of information exchange (*e.g.* patient status, schedule, OR readiness etc.). Dashed arrows represent allowable phone communication between teams on the theme of *patient status* only. The direction of the arrow indicates the receiving end of the phone communication.

5.4.2 Predictions

Predictions were defined based on the interactional model and on known breakdown-related communications and patterns. The two types of predictions – for *breakdown state* and for *normal state* – are elaborated separately below. The notation is introduced in Table 23 and the abbreviations in Table 24.

Table 23. Notation

Symbol	Meaning
↔	Communication between two teams that is bi-directional – it can originate from either team
→	Communication between two teams that is uni-directional – it originates from the team specified at the origin of the arrow, and the team at the tip or the arrow is a recipient of the communication
[X]	The square brackets surround a team specification, in this case team X.
[X : p]	"p" defines a specific information type for the communication. The implication is that no other information type is allowed through the definition of the respective communication
[X: ¬ p]	" ¬ " denotes excepted cases and is equivalent to a logical NOT. The notation is used to signify that all types of information exchange are allowed *except p*.
and	Logical AND – values on both sides should be true in order for the prediction to return true.

Table 24. Abbreviations

Abbreviation	Meaning
PT STATE	Patient state
PT INFO	Patient information
ADM	Admission team
EPR	Electronic patient record system
HA	Holding team (HA=Holding Area)
BR	Block/Anesthesia team (BR = Block room)
OR	Operating room team
OUTpt status	Outpatient status
INpt status	Inpatient status

Next, the set of *normal state* and *breakdown state* predictions are presented.

Normal state

The *normal state* predictions were derived from the interactional models (see Section 5.4.1) by directly translating the information flows into notational expressions. The complete set of predictions is presented in Table 26.

Breakdown state

Known expectations of a *breakdown state* were compiled – the entire set consists of the predictions set forth in Table 25, in addition to the following:

- All calls about PT STATE
- All calls about SCHEDULE
- No answer to a phone call – *i.e.* CONTACTABILITY breakdown
- [ADM] using the EPR system

Table 25 also includes known patterns of coordination indicating a breakdown.

Table 25. Information flow predictions for a *breakdown* state.

	Hospital_1, Phase_1	Hospital_1, Phase_2	Hospital_2
	[Pharmacy] ↔ [ADM]	[Pharmacy] ↔ [ADM]	[Pharmacy] ↔ [ADM]
	[Labs] ↔ [ADM]	[Labs] ↔ [ADM]	[Labs] ↔ [ADM]
	[Post op] ↔ [ADM]	[Post op] ↔ [ADM]	[Post op] ↔ [ADM]
	[Imaging] → [OR desk]	[Imaging] → [OR desk]	[Imaging] → [OR desk]
	[Inpatient floor] → [OR desk]	[Inpatient floor] → [OR desk]	[Inpatient floor] → [OR desk]
	[Post op] → [OR desk]	[Post op] → [OR desk]	[Post op] → [OR desk]
	[OR desk] → [Booking]	[OR desk] → [Booking]	[OR desk] → [Booking]
	[OR desk] → [Maintenance]	[OR desk] → [Maintenance]	[OR desk] → [Maintenance]
	[BR: schedule] → [OR desk]	[BR: schedule] → [OR desk]	[BR: schedule] → [OR desk]
	[OR desk: ¬ pt status] → [BR]	[OR desk: ¬ pt status] → [BR]	[OR desk] → [ICU], except for first call of the day
	[OR desk: ¬ pt status] → [OR]	[OR desk: ¬ pt status] → [OR]	[OR desk] → [Recovery], except for first call of the day
	[ADM: ¬ pt status] → [OR desk]	[ADM] → [OR desk]	[ADM] → [OR]
	[ADM] → [OR]	[OR desk] → [ADM]	[ADM] → [BR]
	[HA] → [OR]	[OR desk] → [Reception]	[OR desk: ¬ staffing] → [OR]
		[ADM] → [OR]	[OR desk] → [BR]
		[HA] → [OR]	[BR: schedule] → [ADM]
			[HA: ¬OR status] → [OR]
Pattern	In any sequence, at least three of these calls are placed: [OR desk] → [ADM] [OR desk] → [HA] [OR desk] → [OR] [OR desk] → [BR] [OR desk] → [Post op] [OR desk] → [Inpatient Floor] [OR desk: page] → [Charge Nurse] [Charge Nurse] → [OR desk]	In any sequence, at least three of these calls are placed: [OR desk] → [ADM] [OR desk] → [HA] [OR desk] → [OR] [OR desk] → [BR] [OR desk] → [Post op] [OR desk] → [Inpatient Floor] [OR desk: page] → [Charge Nurse] [Charge Nurse] → [OR desk]	[TRAUMA: page] → [OR desk] [OR desk] → [TRAUMA] [OR desk] → [OR] [OR desk] → [Anesthesia]

Table 26. Information flow predictions for a *normal* state.

	Hospital_1, Phase_1	Hospital_1, Phase_2	Hospital_2
Reception	[Reception: pt status] → [OR desk]		
Admission [ADM]	[ADM] → [Imaging] [ADM: pt status] → [OR desk]	[ADM] → [Imaging]	
Imaging	[Imaging: pt status] → [ADM]	[Imaging: pt status] → [ADM]	[Imaging: pt status] → [ADM]
Holding [HA]	[HA: pt status] → [OR desk] [HA: pt status] → [BR]	[HA: pt status] → [BR]	[HA: pt status] → [ADM] [HA: OR status] → [OR]
OR desk	[OR desk] → [Reception] [OR desk] → [ADM] [OR desk] → [HA] [OR desk: pt status] → [OR] [OR desk: pt status] → [BR] [OR desk] → [Post op]	[OR desk] → [HA] [OR desk: pt status] → [OR] [OR desk: pt status] → [BR] [OR desk] → [Post op]	[OR desk: pt status] → [Inpatient Floor] [OR desk: staffing] → [OR]
Block Room [BR]	[BR: pt status] → [OR desk] [BR: pt status] → [OR] [BR: OR status] → [OR]	[BR: pt status] → [OR desk] [BR: pt status] → [OR] [BR: OR status] → [OR]	[BR: pt status] → [ADM] [BR: OR status] → [OR]
Operating Room [OR]	[OR] → [OR desk] [OR] → [BR] [OR: pt status] → [HA]	[OR] → [OR desk] [OR] → [BR] [OR: pt status] → [HA]	[OR: INpt status] → [OR desk] [OR: pt status] → [BR] [OR: OUTpt status] → [HA]

Table 27. Coordination properties predicting a breakdown.

Hospital_1, Phase_1	Hospital_1, Phase_2	Hospital_2
PT INFO and TANGIBLE PT STATUS and INTANGIBLE EQUIPMENT and TANGIBLE TANGIBLE and INFO PUSH INTANGIBLE and INFO PULL EQUIPMENT and INFO PUSH PT INFO and INFO PUSH PT STATUS and INFO PULL HUMAN FACTOR and INFO PULL		
DYNAMIC CONDITION and INFO PUSH	DYNAMIC CONDITION and INFO PUSH	PATIENT CARE and INTANGIBLE

Secondary detection: coordination properties

The present research found that properties of coordination and repair of a breakdown are related. These relationships were encapsulated into predictions. Given that the relationships established in this work pertained to breakdowns, the predictions are set to determine the presence of a potential *breakdown state*. When a cross check of two predicted properties returns true, the communication event is deemed to be a breakdown. The full set of coordination properties predictions is shown in Table 27.

5.4.3 Detection procedure

The event logs from the observational data sets for both hospitals were examined with respect to the prediction sets described above. Because the predictions concern only incoming and outgoing calls, and usage of the EPR system, only these particular types of events were tested against the predictions. All other types of events, such as use of artifacts and co-located communication, were ignored. The algorithm shown in Figure 26 was applied in order to determine a breakdown.

```
Input: event - an event from the log of all communication
events comprising the empirical data sets for the 2 hospitals.
An event is characterized by origin & target of communication.
Output: TRUE when a breakdown is detected. FALSE otherwise.

//for each event of type "incoming call", "outgoing call" or
"EPR"
if (event = breakdown state prediction)
        return TRUE
else if (event = normal state prediction)
        return FALSE
else if (event = secondary prediction)
        return TRUE
//since no match for normal state was found, predict breakdown
else
        return TRUE
```

Figure 26: Breakdown detection algorithm for the data sets of this study.

The detection level was adjusted by removing predictions from the previously evaluated prediction set, thus reducing the sensitivity of the algorithm. At first the complete prediction set was applied. Next, the breakdown state prediction [ADM] → [OR] was removed from the set and the algorithm was re-applied. For the third iteration, predictions for all types of information flow related to [HA] → [OR] were excluded from the previous prediction set – these included predictions of normal and of breakdown state. Following was the exclusion of all predictions of normal and breakdown state related to [OR desk] → [OR] from the prediction set of the previous iteration. In the final iteration, the secondary predictions of breakdowns state (Table 27) were taken out.

The choice of predictions to be excluded was determined based on knowledge that these specific predictions detected commonly occurring breakdowns and therefore their exclusion would result in reasonable reduction in breakdown detection. The order of exclusion was not of particular importance - one can use the data in Figure 27 to compute performance for a different sequence. Since the method is a binary classifier system with no ordinal, interval or ratio scale associated with the detection variable, no criterion exists to define proper sequence or prediction set size.

As discussed earlier in this chapter, the sensitivity can be increased by adding further predictions. For the purpose of the breakdown method validation, the goal was to test the detection performance with a basic set of predictions.

Certain breakdown repairs entailed multiple phone calls, each of which matched a breakdown prediction. However, no multiple counts were allowed during the application of the method – *i.e.* these detections were marked as belonging to the same breakdown and did not result in duplicate detections (see Section 5.6.2).

5.4.4 ROC curve evaluation of breakdown detection

To validate the performance of the breakdown detection method, a ROC curve analysis was performed. The application of the algorithm allowed the computation of the TPR and FPR at varying sensitivity levels. The total sample of true positive cases and true negative cases in the three data sets was counted. The true positive sample represents all the actual breakdowns in the data. The true negative sample represents the rest of the recorded events in the data – *i.e.* non-breakdown events. The TPR was computed as the fraction of the true positives output by the detection algorithm in the true positive sample. Likewise, the FPR was determined as the fraction of false positives output by the algorithm in the true negative sample. The TPR range for the full set of predictions was between 95.6% and 97.8%, and the FPR range was between 0.5% and 2.2%. At the lowest sensitivity level, when the predictions described in Section 5.4.3 were all excluded, the TPR range was between 32.4% and 79.5%, and the FPR range was between 0.2% and 0.8%. Figure 27 summarizes the validation outcomes.

Total:	True Positive	True Negative			True Positive	True Negative			True Positive	True Negative		
	137	852			161	429			139	585		
Prediction set	Hospital 1, Phase 1				Hospital 1, Phase 2				Hospital 2			
	True Positive	False Positive	**TPR**	**FPR**	True Positive	False Positive	**TPR**	**FPR**	True Positive	False Positive	**TPR**	**FPR**
with all predictions	131	19	**0.9562**	**0.0223**	155	5	**0.9627**	**0.0117**	136	3	**0.9784**	**0.0051**
"SAU->OR" excluded	126	16	**0.9197**	**0.0188**	148	4	**0.9193**	**0.0093**	127	3	**0.9137**	**0.0051**
above and "HA->OR" excluded	114	12	**0.8321**	**0.0141**	142	4	**0.8820**	**0.0093**	112	3	**0.8058**	**0.0051**
above and "OR desk->OR" excluded	92	7	**0.6715**	**0.0082**	132	3	**0.8199**	**0.0070**	93	1	**0.6691**	**0.0017**
above + no secondary detection	83	7	**0.6058**	**0.0082**	128	3	**0.7950**	**0.0070**	45	1	**0.3237**	**0.0017**

Figure 27: Breakdown detection data. The frequency counts represent incoming and outgoing phone calls. True positive rate (TPR) and false positive rate (FPR) reflect the ratio of detection to actual total sample in the given category (total true positive or true negative, respectively).

The three curves in Figure 28 show the breakdown detection method performance over the three sets of data, with each curve depicting one set. There is high similarity in the outcomes, with slightly better performance for the data from Hospital_2. The lower number of false positives for Hospital_2 reflects the reactive, rather than proactive, culture of information exchange at Hospital_2 – phone calls are most often placed when there is a specific need to acquire information. In contrast, Hospital_1's culture of information exchange at the surgical unit is one of proactive pre-emptive information push that is not associated with a specific breakdown-triggered need. Therefore, the potential for the algorithm to detect false positives is increased. In Phase 2 (Hospital_1), the overall phone communication is slightly reduced as a result of the introduction of the eWhiteboard as a communication tool. At the same time the culture of proactive pre-emptive information exchange is preserved – the result is a lowered opportunity for false positive detections and therefore a slightly better algorithm performance.

The area under the curve (AUC) as a standard performance measure shows very high values for all three datasets, ranging from 0.971 to 0.987. These values demonstrate an excellent performance achieved in detecting inter-team breakdowns in the two hospitals through the application of the breakdown detection method.

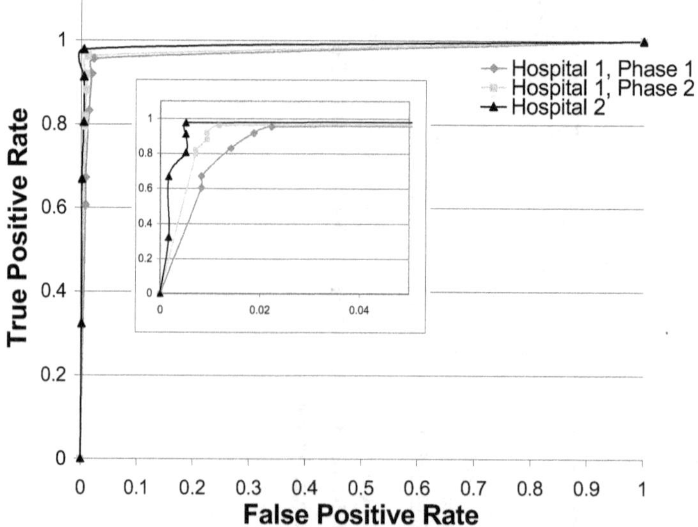

Figure 28: ROC curve for breakdown detection method over the three sets of data. The area under the curve (AUC) for Hospital_1 Phase 1 is 0.971, for Hospital_1 Phase 2 is 0.977, and for Hospital_2 is 0.987.

5.5 Discussion

The breakdown detection method proposed in this chapter was applied and validated over the data coming from the three empirical studies in two hospitals. The evaluation of the method revealed excellent breakdown detection performance, even with a basic set of predictions that focused on phone communication only. Inter-team coordination breakdowns were correctly identified 95.6%-97.8% of the time with the initial set of predictions. After iteratively reducing the level of sensitivity of the algorithm, breakdown detection was between 32.4% and 79.5% at the lowest sensitivity level tested. At all sensitivity levels, the false positive rate remained very low – between 0.2% and 2.2%. These results clearly indicate that the breakdown detection method provides meaningful and correct outcomes. Furthermore, the false negatives (FNR) - *i.e.* missed breakdowns, are more critical when it comes to addressing safety issues than the false positives – the tolerance for missing the detection of breakdowns in safety-critical applications should be minimized. Thus, the very high TPR exhibited by the breakdown detection method, reflecting low rate of false negatives (FNR + TPR = 1), is of utmost importance and makes it especially suitable for applications seeking to address safety issues. Although the detection rate is dependent on the scope of the predictions – the more predictions, the higher the detection rate – the results of the validation proved that even with a moderate scope of predictions limited to the analysis of phone communication only, the breakdown detection method performs very well.

The breakdown detection method would best be utilized in the facilitation and evaluation of safety and process improvement interventions, including technology implementations. The detection method would be applied to determine the pre-intervention state of affairs with respect to a particular problem – *i.e.* a single type of breakdown such as patient consent issues. The output would provide a baseline for the evaluation of the intervention. After implementation, the breakdown detection method would be re-applied to measure the outcome of the intervention with a modified prediction set to reflect the new information flow trajectories expected of breakdown-free information exchange in the surgical unit. The post-intervention breakdown detection would provide an accurate assessment of the most current state of affairs as compared to pre-implementation. As the adoption study in this book showed, clinical performance measures used in the evaluation of process improvement endeavors, such as the introduction of the eWhiteboard as an inter-team communication tool, do not reflect the persistent communication issues that remain past implementation and undermine success.

The breakdown detection method is particularly useful because of the minimal cost associated with its application. First, the information flow is commonly formally defined within each organization and unit and thus can be obtained without the high cost of analysis. Another non-expensive option for information flow mapping is to interview clinicians in each micro-system. Second, this study demonstrated that the method can be effectively and successfully applied without the need for investment in analysis or monitoring technology. With current telephone technology in place in most Western hospitals, call tracking/logging could be utilized without any expense. These technologies will further reduce the cost associated with observer data collection. The only consideration in using telephone logs is to find a way to determine the foci/theme of coordination of phone communication. Otherwise, the method would still detect breakdowns, but the accuracy will be reduced. Only the secondary detections – those facilitated by cross checking the properties of breakdowns and their repairs, require human analysis capabilities in addition to the pure technical data collection.

Another important advantage of the breakdown detection method is that it provides detection from a global view of the system process under consideration, due to its focus on inter-team coordination. Additionally, in the case of automated inter-team communication monitoring (see Section 5.7), the method would produce a better description of reality than the data coming from manual data collection (as was the case of this study). The latter suffers from the constraint of having a single viewpoint of data collection – an observer is present one place at a time. Thus, the resulting breakdowns view of the activity of the various teams is time-distributed and reflects breakdown rates at dispersed moments in time. When applied by automated means of activity monitoring, such as when outgoing and incoming phone calls are tracked or logged, the breakdown detection method will produce an accurate global view of coordination breakdowns among all collaborating teams at any point in time.

5.6 Limitations of the method

Detecting breakdowns by applying the method proposed in this chapter poses several challenges – some breakdowns cannot be detected, others produce duplicates, and certain culturally related communication behaviors result in false positives. This section will detail such problems identified during the validation of the method and discuss their implications.

5.6.1 False Negatives

When a breakdown repair is executed at the same physical location as the one where the breakdown was detected, the method as applied in this study would produce a false negative (*i.e.* it would miss the breakdown). Although not frequent, there were several cases of such situations in our data. A solution to the issue of false negatives is the utilization of more advanced context-aware technology such as location-aware sensors (see Section 5.7). The trade-off for improved accuracy in breakdown detection is the required investment in sensor technology. However, depending on the specific needs and goals for which the breakdown detection method is used, such an investment may be justified, such as when serious safety issues are suspected.

Another occasion when false negatives were identified during the breakdown detection method validation was for cases when no action of repair was taken from the person who detected the breakdown. The issue of false negatives in this scenario is a consequence of the fact that the method was applied over observational data. This data, as discussed earlier, is subject to the limitation of a single viewpoint at a given instance in time. Assuming that a repair will be undertaken by some team at some moment in time, the breakdown will be detected if several observers collect data simultaneously at different team locations or if automated phone tracking/logging is implemented.

5.6.2 Duplicate true positives

Breakdown repair work is sometimes distributed through time and executed in parallel to other coordination activities. Specifically, this situation applies to breakdowns that cannot be resolved immediately and require follow-up repair efforts. In its basic form, the breakdown detection method would not recognize repair work efforts that are scattered across time, and interleaved with other coordination work, as relevant to a single breakdown. The result is the output of several true positives for a single breakdown. The duplicate positives can be eliminated by a higher degree of sophistication of the algorithm. Alternatively, they can be tolerated and treated as data noise – there were only several such instances in our data. In any case, the overall picture produced by the breakdown detection method still has a high degree of accuracy and is a good reflection of actual breakdown rates.

5.6.3 False positives

The perioperative process is a safety-critical environment where, as in other safety-critical domains, a degree of redundancy is highly valued as service to reliability and resilience of operations. The level and degree of formality of redundancy can vary from hospital to hospital. *All of the false positives* produced by our data sets from both hospitals, were due to either duplication of effort or pre-emptive inter-team information exchange, especially during low workload periods. These inter-team communications stem from the goal to maintain reliability and resilience. For example, when a nurse in Admissions noticed an unusual procedure listed on the consent form, she called the surgeon to alert him/her to that fact. Another common occurrence in the false positives data was when the OR finished a surgery prior to scheduled completion time, they would call the Admissions team to inform them so that later scheduled patients can be prepared earlier than planned. Similarly, the Holding and Admissions teams sometimes called the OR to check the status of the current surgery so they can plan their local patient care activities. Occasionally, during low workload times, clinicians would call the OR desk to pre-emptively check if there are any changes to the schedule. All of these situations resulted in false positives.

Our data shows a higher degree of false positives at Hospital_1 (Figure 27). The numbers correctly reflect the difference in organizational communication culture - at Hospital_1 it was one of proactive information pushing, while at Hospital_2 it was one of reactive information pulling per need. Hence, the greater number of false positives for Hospital_1.

5.7 Automated detection

Data collection, extraction and analysis are major methodological challenges in empirical qualitative research [310]. Both have an extremely high cost as transcription and coding are labor intensive. Correlating data becomes cumbersome because it triggers numerous iterations or re-coding. Automated data collection would reduce the efforts of both transcription and extraction, and facilitate the automated detection of breakdown with minimal cost.

There are two ways that automated breakdown detection is envisioned with the proposed method. As discussed earlier, current phone technology utilized in hospitals in most of the world already log incoming and outgoing phone communications. The logs can be acquired and used as transcripts for retroactive breakdown detection with the method. Additionally, simple software applications can be coded to automatically monitor the phone logging process in real time, to write breakdown detections to a file, and to analyze them.

Another option for automated data collection, extraction and ultimately breakdown detection is through the utilization of context and/or location aware sensors, such as RFID technology. People and asset trajectories are easily identifiable with RFID data, as well as trajectory intersections. Thus, the approach can be considered in tandem with phone call monitoring in order to improve detection accuracy rate (*i.e.* the issue of false negatives due to repair efforts taking place in the same location as the detection). RFID data coming from staff ID badges can be monitored to identify situations when clinicians from different teams are in close physical proximity within the same physical space – if breakdown predictions for *normal state* do not include an expectation for such inter-team proximity, a potential breakdown would be detected.

Telephone and RFID data can reduce the total cost of breakdown detection and increase accuracy of detection. Both technologies are implemented in many hospitals around the world to seamlessly provide information used to improve healthcare operations. In such hospitals there will be no setup-cost associated with their use.

5.8 Chapter summary

The method proposed in this chapter provides an efficient and inexpensive approach to the detection of inter-team coordination breakdowns in the surgical unit operations. Given the rise in evidence that such breakdowns are often a consequence to technological implementations, and the precursors to safety hazards, being able to assess their presence pre- and post-implementation is crucial.

The breakdown detection method is the first step required for breakdown management within the context of the daily operations of surgical units. By mapping information flow expectations for the different information needs of clinical work – such as patient status information flow, schedule status information flow, staffing coordination information flow, etc. – an analyst can derive a set of predictions that serve as input to the algorithm for detecting the breakdowns. The algorithm is based on the notion that behaviors that do not comply with predictions of normal information flow are potential breakdowns. The algorithm can be augmented to include predictions of communication behaviors that indicate the presence of breakdowns. The method was verified over the data from the observational studies of this work (Phases 1 & 2 in Hospital_1, and the data from Hospital_2) and demonstrated excellent detection performance.

The breakdown detection method allows an analyst to determine the amount of breakdowns for different types of breakdowns, before and after technology or intervention implementations. The next chapter will develop the second step in the management of breakdowns - the strategies for system design to aid improvement efforts and the prevention of breakdowns. By re-applying the breakdown detection method following an improvement intervention, one can evaluate the success in terms of reduced or persistent presence of breakdowns.

6

Breakdown management

This chapter materializes the knowledge on breakdowns acquired in this research into design recommendations and establishes a blueprint for future work in the management of breakdowns in the perioperative setting. The chapter begins with a presentation of a set of guidelines and a system design framework for breakdown management that are tailored to the requirements of the surgical domain. Next, current challenges in breakdown management are identified and directions for future work are defined.

Given that coordination breakdowns have a significant impact on both patient safety and on surgical system performance, what can be done to prevent or minimize their effect? What are the general strategies, independent of specific errors, that can lead the way to inter-team coordination improvement? This chapter aims to answer the aforementioned questions by providing guidelines for system design that capitalize on the understanding of breakdowns and related coordination mechanisms acquired through this work. The guidelines are then integrated into a system design framework that also incorporates the breakdown detection method as a tool for assessment of the severity of breakdowns in everyday work. The chapter concludes by laying out the agenda for future work on breakdown management in the perioperative field.

6.1 System design for the perioperative setting

6.1.1 Guidelines for process and technology (re-)design

A number of researchers suggest innovative technological solutions such as eWhiteBoards, context-aware systems, and sensor technologies [39, 243, 305] as solutions to coordination and communication breakdowns in healthcare. Several guidelines for design have also been proposed [59, 121]. This section shifts the focus to the methodological space. Based on the findings of this study design guidelines are proposed for the early stages of system design. Next, a design framework is suggested that adapts current system development lifecycle activities by integrating the guidelines.

The research reported in this book showed that the majority of breakdowns in surgical patient care are relevant to the inter-team dimension – *i.e.* they pertain to communication processes and information exchange between micro-systems. Breakdowns were found to propagate downstream in the process of surgical care, passing through micro-system interfaces until detected and addressed, which increases their repair cost proportionately to the propagation distance. The cost of breakdown repair has implications not only for the amount of incurred communication overhead, but also for the amount of interruptions produced to clinical work and for safety. Safety was found to be at least partially related to the availability of communication protocols for dealing with breakdowns. The cultural factor of lack of trust at team interfaces was found to be a disabler of successful technology adoption. All of the findings point to serious latent factors related to communication and coordination that lie at team boundaries, at the macro-system level. How can system design address this type of latent factors?

The outcomes of this research correspond to problems other industries have addressed in the past – *e.g.* the aviation, reliability engineering, production and manufacturing, software and systems engineering domains. A detailed review of the ways in which these industries have addressed breakdown management is provided in Appendix D.1. In summary, the approaches adopted in these domains address system-level breakdowns in several ways: through 1) a multidisciplinary approach, 2) a systems perspective, 3) a focus on early prevention and allowing no opportunities for propagation, 4) a balance between procedure compliance and flexibility, and 5) a culture change. Based on the integration of the findings of this study and the above insights from other fields, this section describes specific guidelines for process and technology design tailored to the perioperative domain so that breakdowns be minimized. The guidelines do not address culture change as this issues was not covered by findings of this work. The guidelines are informed by the approaches in the other domains but are not dependent on specific techniques. Techniques are only suggested as examples of tools that may be appropriate. The target implementation of the guidelines is the initial stages of system design – during task and workflow analysis at the requirements stage. At the core of the guidelines is the notion to seek information needs and potential breakdowns at the systems level, rather than to look only for person-oriented human errors. A design framework integrating the guidelines follows their description.

Process analysis guidelines

(I) Mind the entire process workflow, not only the problem taskflow. This research showed that most breakdowns relate to inter-team coordination. The particular problem that a redesigned procedure or a piece of technology is to support should be positioned with respect to the entire process, not just the immediate environment of the user. All micro-systems within the process, their inputs and outputs should be analyzed, regardless of the apparent relevance to the issue at hand. Information and tasks that seem pertinent to specific segments or people in the process can have unobtrusive implicit relevance to other parts of the socio-technical system. Hospitals are fragmented systems. This study confirmed that breakdowns in care delivery may derive from factors further upstream and distant within the network of a hospital's organizational processes. Asking users to clarify inputs and outputs to their task is not sufficient. A designer should deliberate the entire system process to build confidence that all inter-team requirements are identified, including those subtle processes that are carried over implicit coordination mediums. Although a procedure or computational solution is to support a micro level problem (i.e. scheduling ORs), analysis should address the effect that the new application will have at the macro level – on the entire perioperative system. Concern-oriented approaches to systems engineering [143]

can be particularly relevant in addressing system level requirements, as long as the minimum set of stakeholders is extended to include representatives of the entire target user population, as opposed to the subset of direct end-users.

For example, designing an OR scheduling system should not only consider the scheduling-related tasks and users, but the entire perioperative macro-system, with verification of inputs and outputs – those related to scheduling and those that might not seem relevant at first sight. Nurses in surgical pre-admission and in admission might not be direct users of such a scheduling system, but the system state is extremely relevant to their work.

(II) Consider coordination themes with respect to process. Provide efficient means for repair from breakdowns. The analysis of breakdowns in this research study revealed that the organizational process and coordination theme determine the repair strategy. Although there may be variations in instantiation, the basic structure of the perioperative system process and the themes of coordination are common across settings. Thus, coordination solutions to be embedded in new procedures or technology should be designed with consideration of coordination themes and surgical process, where for each theme appropriate information means are provided. The thematic breakdowns resolved with information pull can be relieved by means of information push so as to eliminate the need for pulling. The thematic breakdowns resolved with information push can benefit from enhanced communication channels between parties that minimize the cost associated with repair. For instance, patient information breakdowns are predominantly resolved via information push (because the task of providing the missing patient information is usually delegated to the responsible person). An efficient channel of 'push' communication for patient information breakdown repair delegation can be a motion scan of the respective form's barcode, or a read of its RFID tag, with a dedicated reader that sends a request for the missing information to the relevant responsible party for the given information type.

(III) Embed barriers in the system that prevent breakdown propagation, or consider re-engineering the process. This research showed that the length of travel of a breakdown through the system determines the repair cost. Therefore, the goal of design should be to minimize, even eliminate, the distance that breakdowns can propagate in order to reduce the repair cost and associated interruptions and safety implications. To this end, the completeness of all inputs to the socio-technical micro-systems (both operational and IT-inputs) should be verified against the outputs of the preceding process step. In essence, the accuracy and completeness of communication interfaces between teams must be verified before clinical work is allowed to proceed. Design barriers should be embedded at each surgical patient care transition, thus preventing the progression of flow upon

missing inputs. Immunity to breakdown propagation should be a system design requirement. Failure propagation modeling can be utilized through techniques such as Failure Mode and Effects Analysis (FMEA) and Advanced Cause Consequence Analysis (ACCA), with a focus on information needs, to support work with breakdown management design. While disablers of breakdown propagation should be placed as far from the actual surgery as possible, some flexibility can be introduced – *e.g.* though multiple information flow trajectories. In some cases, re-engineering the process will be more reasonable in allowing for inherent flexibility and safety than introducing additional barriers.

To prevent halts in the perioperative system (an undesirable effect of enforcement of the system inputs), barriers should be implemented with caution and with a degree of flexibility by means of an explicit timeframe or system boundary - pre-emptive reminders could first warn of outstanding inputs, and 'soft' IT-system halts could be explored as subsequent more intrusive interventions. For example, if reminders to acquire patient allergy information did not result in data input for the allergy field of the patient record up until 24 hours prior to surgery, the application view for the functional role responsible for coordination of patient information can simulate a halt at an appropriate time (not in the middle of the user's task). This would mean a freeze for several seconds with a display of the particular patient record and appropriate message that this patient's missing information will produce a surgery halt. The user should be able to 'unfreeze' the application after several seconds, or to delegate responsibility for the record to another functional role with an explicit digital handshake. While such a solution would incur minimal human resource cost at the local level, since breakdown propagation will be reduced, the overall communication cost associated with breakdown repair will be minimized.

(IV) Mind tangibility – it is important to users. The findings of this research showed that tangibility is relevant to the coordination theme and determines the choice of repair strategy. The design of coordination solutions should account for the tangibility requirements of coordination processes as per their theme and should provide the relevant push/pull means to facilitate the information transfer. For example, patient information will always relate to the tangible and therefore can continue being supported by tangible artifacts – the effort should be in improving the information presentation. Patient care issues, on the other hand, relate to the intangible which affords greater opportunity for breakdowns in a distributed teams environment. This research found that most tangible-related breakdowns are resolved by pushing information, while most intangible-based breakdowns trigger information pull. Therefore, intangible-based breakdowns will best be supported via seamless communication devices that allow on-time

coordination negotiation, information pull and efficient breakdown repair, without the constraints of traditional telephones and intercoms that require a clinician to cross a room, lookup a number, dial, and stay stationary for the duration of the negotiation. Voice-operated badges [36] are an existing communication solution that can support coordination related to the intangible in an efficient and transparent manner.

(V) Consider cultural factors. The technology adoption study found that lack of trust at inter-team boundaries is a disabler to successful coordination improvement efforts. The problem can be addressed by the design of coordination solutions that promote trust. The design should involve all teams, through a discussion of their respective needs and expectations of each other. Solutions should be generated and re-designed through continuous discussions until all teams adopt the evolved intervention with confidence that it serves their information needs, which translates into behaviors that speak to that effect.

(VI) Examine recurrent patterns of coordination. This research established that recurrent patterns of coordination are present in surgical care work. These patterns of coordination are informal solutions to recurrent breakdowns. The coordination structures comprising these patterns are easily detectable observable behaviors and are good targets for efficiency improvement efforts. Clinicians can benefit tremendously from offloading these recurrent communications through more automated technological means.

(VII) Examine recurrent breakdowns. This research showed that the existence of communication protocol for re-coordination upon a breakdown can make a significant difference in the potential for the breakdown to affect patient safety. Recurrent breakdowns that are not associated with a coordination solution are a prime target for communication protocol or technological solution.

Task analysis guidelines

A qualitative approach, in combination with a formal description of activity, is required for an early and feasible solution of safety threats in high-risk clinical system design. Other safety-critical fields such as military and aerospace use qualitative design methodologies based on human error and risk analysis. Such methods incorporate erroneous user actions analysis into the task models [33, 94, 224, 231]. Classification schemes of human error in system interaction help streamline error predictions [137, 234, 238]. The MECHA method [94], guidewords-based techniques [224], and the THEA technique [231] analyze erroneous user actions - cognitive and behavioral, i.e. slips, lapses and mistakes (a.k.a. skill-, rule- and knowledge-based errors). However, for clinical contexts these methods have too narrow a scope of analysis – they are human-centered but not process-oriented. They focus only on an individual's potential to err, at the cognitive and behavioral levels, while cooperative aspects predisposing breakdown situations are neglected. The design of surgical care procedures or computational applications should also consider communication and coordination breakdowns, computational communication breakdowns, and external workflow influences.

(VIII) Integrate task model, system model and workflow model into a coherent Cooperative Surgical Activity Model (CSAM). This research showed evidence that latent communication factors lie at all system levels – the task, the workflow, and the macro-system. A task model should therefore be able to reflect the complexity of clinical work and allow for analysis of the full range of communication, coordination and other issues that can arise from introducing a new procedure or technology into an existing clinical context. To that end, the level of analysis should include a balanced integration of user task model, technical system communication interfaces (human interface and system-system interface with appropriate state instances), and workflow model. While the main focus remains the specific task and associated user actions, the relevant technical system interactions and relevant workflow relationships to other activities and organizational factors are necessary information sources for a complete task analysis. Peripheral systems, people, objects, tools and data sources should be reflected in the model.

(IX) Focus on joint activity processes – localization of communication and coordination hotspots. This research revealed the importance of communication and coordination activities to clinical work. In the CSAM, particular attention should be paid to reflect and analyze the implications of all participatory actions of agents derived from each individual user's task model (i.e. each functional role). The model should reflect all actions that contribute to coordination of the activity.

(X) Represent technology in the task model – localization of human-computer interaction and system-system interaction hotspots. The present research and previous work have shown that technical and equipment failures are common in the perioperative setting. The role of technology as an interactor [32] in the perioperative activity is as significant as that of humans – when a system fails the safety-related consequences could be as severe as those of a physician being unavailable at a time of emergency. The CSAM should incorporate relevant communication interfaces from the technical system model, including the respective parameters and system states.

(XI) Design for safety through breakdowns analysis. This research demonstrated the significant impact of breakdowns on surgical operations and on safety. Safety is the property of the interrelationships and interconnections between parts of a

socio-technical system [94]. Thus, analysis should focus on identifying those interrelationships and interconnections that can produce breakdowns and challenge the safety of the socio-technical system. This implies a thorough analysis of user actions, human-computer and system-system interactions that can produce human error or communication and coordination breakdowns. The temporal aspects of the interrelationships and interconnections among actions are of specific importance to correctly identify the conditions that will lead the system to an unsafe state (Breakdowns analysis is elaborated on later in this chapter).

(XII) Either entirely replace a repair/coordination structure, or keep it intact. In this study, a number of coordination repair structures were observed in the perioperative setting. Similar to personal behavioral modules in the field of Psychology, repair structures can be conceptualized as joint activity-related behavioral modules. As such, they can be replaced by IT solutions as an entity, but should not be segmented (*i.e.* with only certain segments being automated). The entire action sequence must be automated. Otherwise, conditions predisposing to human error and breakdowns are created [288].

Breakdowns analysis guidelines

This section suggests how potential breakdowns can be anticipated by thoroughly examining the task and process models for the clinical activity under consideration. The exploration of breakdowns during workflow and task analysis must look at activity as comprised of agents' work on three analytical levels: the activity space, the problem space, and the action space (Figure 29). *Actions* can be individual and participatory (i.e. individual actions that are coordinated with other people in the activity and intended to be part of the joint activity) [54]. Actions are subject to cognitive and behavioral errors. Participatory actions make up the work in the *activity space* - negotiation of goals, plans, procedures, etc. These are needed to organize the task and are part of the system work. Thus, work in the activity space is susceptible to coordination breakdowns. The *problem space* is made of both types of actions – it reflects individual and joint work on the problem-solving of the medical problem. Work in this area is vulnerable to communication breakdowns. Given that the *activity* and *problem spaces* subsume *actions*, cognitive and behavioral errors can propagate to communication and coordination breakdowns. Technology is present on two levels of breakdown analysis in the activity - as an interactor through its user interface it allows for use errors; and as a mediator through its system interface it allows for communication breakdowns at the computational level.

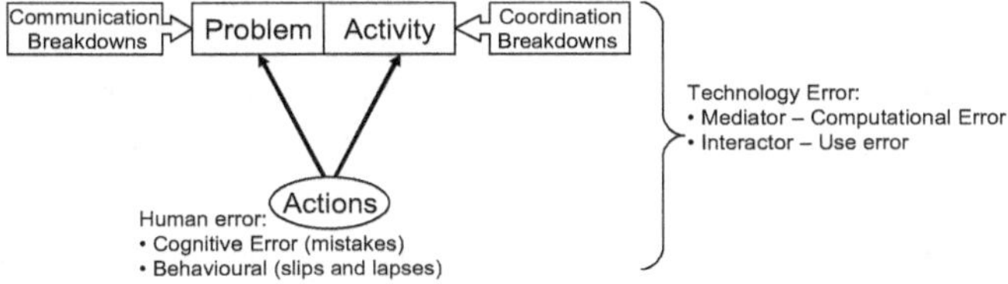

Figure 29. Analyzing surgical work from a joint activity perspective, including the errors and breakdowns each type of participant work is prone to.

Once a task model is created, it is traversed from low-level actions to higher-level tasks and the full range of potential errors and breakdowns are analyzed for each action in the tree. The possible human error and breakdown patterns considered are: *cognitive* and *behavioral* errors, *coordination breakdowns*, *communication breakdowns*, *system-as-mediator* and *system-as-interactor* errors. Classification schemes are used and techniques applied for human error analysis. The inputs to both human error and breakdowns analysis are: envisioned error scenarios and application specialists' feedback (require domain knowledge); observations, incident and accident reports, historical and empirical data, and other technologies' specifications (objective points of reference). Temporal factors influence the occurrences of errors and breakdowns and should be considered: what is the time safety threshold for each task (e.g. 3 seconds vs. 5 minutes). The time and space configuration of the task – same place/different place/same time/different time – should be exploited in the breakdowns analysis. Lastly, each predicted failure is associated with an outcome, and risk analysis is performed.

6.1.2 System design framework

This section proposes a system design framework tailored to perioperative work. The framework integrates the knowledge acquired through this study and positions the design guidelines (suggested earlier in this chapter) in the context of the system design lifecycle by adapting some of the development activities. The framework extends traditional user-centered design approaches currently used for the design of medical technology, such as [4, 6, 190, 208, 209], to include coordination processes and breakdowns at the macro level through a systems approach. The framework targets the design and development of interventions such as procedures, processes and technology to address communication and coordination breakdowns in surgical patient care. This framework is relevant to the initial stages of system design and throughout the development cycle.

1. Requirements gathering – follow guideline *(I)* – elicit needs from all stakeholders in the surgical process, including those that are not envisioned to be the procedure or technology users. Employ formal IT-system description methods considering all stakeholders (e.g. ANSI/IEEE 1471[143]) to derive a complete set of requirements that addresses direct and indirect user needs in addition to the minimum set of stakeholder concerns. Probe for a thorough understanding of the domain system processes, not only the particular design task problem.

2. Detect breakdowns – apply the breakdown detection method to identify the occurrence of breakdowns and to establish a baseline for evaluation of the design effort. The output from the breakdown detection method is used as input to the design of breakdown disablers.

3. Task and workflow analysis – both should address domain system level processes of coordination, implicit and explicit, tangible and intangible. Guidelines *(II)*, *(IV)*, *(VIII-X)*, and *(XII)* should be applied. Existing concern-oriented techniques [253] can facilitate the identification of cross-disciplinary task and workflow-related requirements. The task and workflow models can be integrated into a CSAM.

4. Breakdowns analysis – examine the breakdowns that are recurrent and produce most overhead, and analyze the underlying reasons that are responsible for the occurrence of breakdowns – *e.g.* inadequate procedures, culture, incompatible goals between teams, etc. Participation of all stakeholders and multidisciplinary experts at this step is essential. Guidelines *(V-VII)*, *(XI)*, and the *breakdown analysis guidelines* are relevant.

5. Concept design – address the effects of the new procedure or IT-system on the macro level processes identified in the previous steps. Consider between embedding new barriers or re-engineering of the process. Follow guideline *(III)*.

6. Envisioned task and workflow analysis – similar to step 3, address system level processes and the considerations outlined in guidelines *(II)*, *(IV)*, *(VIII-X)*, and *(XII)*. Future task and workflow impact are verified with the entire target user population, at the inter-professional and inter-team levels, through existing techniques [253].

7. Human error analysis over envisioned task flow and workflows - as in other safety-critical domains [33, 94, 224, 231].

8. Breakdowns analysis over envisioned task flow and workflows – the full range of potential breakdowns is explored – techniques of predictive breakdown analysis should be employed, such as those described in [271] and in [102]. Probabilistic failure propagation modeling can be utilized through techniques such as FMEA and ACCA to facilitate design decisions. Validation from all stakeholders and participation of multidisciplinary experts at this step is essential.

Guidelines *(V-VII), (XI),* and the *breakdown analysis guidelines* are relevant.

9. Mapping of predicted failures to anticipated adverse outcomes and risk analysis execution, as in [145].

10. Analysis of contextual factors.

11. Design solutions – inform solutions based on the above analyses; provide appropriate information means based on process and coordination theme - as in guideline *(II)*; embed barriers to prevent breakdown propagation – as in guideline *(III)*; provide suitable tangibility interactions based on coordination theme – as in guideline *(IV)*; consider the solution in the context of the organizational culture – as in guideline *(V)*, and mind human factors – as in guideline *(XII)*.

12. Early system prototyping or procedure training, followed by implementation.

13. Breakdown detection and evaluation testing – apply the breakdown detection method to identify the occurrence of breakdowns and to compare with the baseline. If improvement is not absolutely successful, re-iterate the design effort until the solution evolves to a more mature design.

14. Keep an eye on adoption – continuous monitoring over time and openness to solution re-design are key to ensuring efficiency, safety and complete integration.

6.1.3 Discussion

The design guidelines are supplementary to traditional techniques currently utilized for user task, workflow and requirements analysis (e.g. focus groups, interviews, questionnaires, scenarios, use-cases, etc.). The recommendations integrate the approaches adopted in other industries to address breakdown management with the findings from this research that are specific to the perioperative environment. The resulting guidelines and system design framework for the management of breakdowns are prescriptive of types of analyses to be undertaken in the quest to address system level latent factors of communication and coordination, but are also general enough to allow designers to continue using their preferred techniques of analysis. The guidelines serve to expand the focus of analysis during the early system design stages and to steer it to those issues that are specifically essential to surgical work. The guidelines facilitate the designer's work to adopt an approach that does not fail to address the communication and coordination demands of the perioperative process. The proposed system design framework for breakdown management integrates the knowledge acquired through this study by positioning the guidelines in the context of the system design lifecycle. The framework can be applied during early (re-)design stages, but also can easily be utilized in the context of software integration over existing hospital implementations, as well as in hospital IT infrastructures design. Additionally, some of the recommended analyses can be used to inform technology procurement decisions.

The system design framework for breakdown management in the surgical setting is anticipatory of breakdowns at the individual and system levels. An optimal fit between a process or technology and the intended setting and users is critical for design and successful implementation [140]. Current literature abounds with examples of clinical technologies holding a promise of adoption, efficiency and safety improvement success. However, these technologies often do not meet expectations once integrated into the end-user environment. Indeed, the new technology/procedure often introduces unanticipated problems [160, 247, 319]. While it is impossible to predict every potentially negative consequence in every possible user environment, applying a more holistic and anticipatory analysis framework, like the one proposed here, will minimize the range of procedure or technology integration issues that may occur. Additionally, utilizing the approach from the hospital consumer side (i.e. during procurement and integration) will further increase the return on investment in increased analysis by assuring that the right technology is chosen for a given environment and process. Such holistic, process-oriented analysis is currently non-standard. The framework derived from this study will have significant impact on improving transparency in healthcare technology integration, in enhancing quality and efficiency, and safety.

The idea of minimizing breakdown propagation that underlies some of the guidelines, and drawn on the basis of the findings of this research and of the work in other industries, aims to address not only communication cost reduction, but also to ameliorate conditions of safety hazards. Pushing error detection and prevention upstream translates well into the surgical system due to the linearity of the surgical process. In addition, many of the breakdowns in the surgical setting are due to missing, delayed, unclear, and incomplete information related to surgical preparation work [254] that is the input to patient care on the day of surgery. Therefore, efforts focused on breakdown prevention and detection in the early stages of the surgical process – Patient Referral, Surgeon's Office, Pre-Admission – should reduce a significant amount of the repair cost and the level of latent safety threats. Rigorous efforts in completion of the surgical package (*i.e.* patient chart) from the surgeon's office can help decrease the amount of workload on the day of surgery, as well as the level of uncertainty, need for coordination, and interruptions (i.e. multiplier effects). The work of pre-admission units, where applicable, can further help prevent breakdown propagation by enforcing completeness of the surgical package's auxiliary inputs such as current blood tests, consults, exams, etc. Basically, shifting the main point of breakdown detection and repair from the day of surgery to the micro-systems that precede it is deemed to have significant implications for reducing breakdown impact. While not all breakdowns stem from system inputs, reducing the total of breakdowns on the day of surgery is considered beneficial.

Another positive outlook on the proposed design framework comes from its commonalities with Lean management. In recent years, increasing evidence demonstrates the utility of Lean Management to improving work processes in healthcare organizations. The core of the proposed framework relates closely to the principles of Lean (with the assumption that frontline clinicians are actively involved in design), while applying them to the system design domain. Lean management's fundamental concept is to identify waste and inefficiencies in a process and to create solutions that improve operations to a value-optimal workflow. When applied to healthcare organizations, Lean Management has had positive impact on patient satisfaction, productivity, cost, quality, and efficiency [13, 79]. Breakdowns in healthcare operations that were examined in this research cause a tremendous amount of waste in the process, which is the necessitated repair work. The suggested design framework applies the core principles of Lean management to the design of processes/technology in order to produce a lean technology-supported process - reducing errors, breakdowns and repair overhead results in a lean design of clinical work through the integration of procedural and technological solutions. Both Lean management and the proposed framework design efficiency with an outlook on socio-technical system level processes.

6.1.4 Future directions for work in technology adoption

The issue of trust identified by this work is a social factor not previously reported from studies in the clinical domain. The problem pertains to the domain of organizational culture and deserves a further look. Perhaps greater degree of automation in status communication technologies will avoid trust-related breakdowns. Future technology should aim to ensure the maintenance of reliable operations in a way that ameliorates potential inter-team mistrust. As healthcare IT moves towards technology implementations across the continuum of care, and current legislations are pushing in this direction, such as the HITECH Act and stimulus package in the U.S. for adoption of electronic medical records, the issue of trust will surface more often.

The role of trust in adoption in mediated collaborative work has been studied in other domains such as e-commerce [104] and also falls under the more general problem of User Experience (UX) [123, 169]. Current literature suggests that user-centered design approaches and system performance determine technology adoption. Ease of use and usefulness are the key factors found to predict acceptance [284]. The findings of this study indicate that user-centered approaches to the design of collaborative technologies that support clinical work are not sufficient to produce a successful implementation. There is a tight relation between the "social" and "technical" aspects in a socio-technical system. Successful adoption of a system is significantly influenced by underlying socio-organizational factors in the end-user environment. The challenge such factors present is lack of clear predictability parameters. Designers and users cannot envision the complete impact of system integration. Time and again research studies reveal that understanding the work, the workflow, the context, even the organization, is inadequate in facilitating complete predictability of technology integration. Thus, the importance of adopting a continuous improvement approach becomes paramount in the quest to address such invisible organizational culture factors.

Given the importance of IT to today's surgical operations and the growing number of partial successes with implementations, future work could focus on the development of accurate predictable UX models. These models would focus on the clinical end-user and the socio-organizational factors in their environment. Such models in other domains translate user parameters into product specifications with an outlook on adoption – they have been successful in the manufacturing industry [205]. A retrospective approach to building a UX model may be more appropriate for the surgical domain at this point. Future research should examine factors that represent strong candidate predictors of UX based on existing related studies. In this work, trust was found to be a major contributing factor. In other studies it was the transformation of information from private to public [301, 319], the quality of the connection medium [275], or the shift in power, control and autonomy [25]. In addition, generic adoption parameters like end-user's level of experience with IT, spatial location of technology in-use, institutional turnover rate, etc. should be considered. Being able to accurately predict user experience will be both beneficial to surgical operations and economical from a development point of view.

Lastly, a carefully designed meta-analysis study with data from existing work on technology acceptance in different hospital settings, coupled with sound theoretical frameworks from psychology, sociology and communication science, will shed light on the curious but yet unresolved issue of the discrepancy between the self-reported attitudes and observable behaviors. Insights thus drawn will enable the HCI community to develop more reliable and valid evaluation methods for usability and user experience [168, 248].

6.2 Future perspectives for breakdown management in the surgical setting

This section will briefly review the state of affairs of breakdown management in healthcare so far. Specifically, the section will identify the practices of other domains (identified in Appendix D.1) that have been utilized within the hospital environment. Next, the challenges against existing efforts will be discussed and areas for future work will be identified.

6.2.1 Efforts so far

Recent years have marked a growing recognition in healthcare, and specifically in surgery, of the contribution of latent factors such as coordination breakdowns to preventable adverse events in patient care, including fatalities. Efforts to improve patient safety by addressing the underlying issues have been initiated around the world. The majority of initiatives have turned for insights to aviation as it is a safety-critical field and offers years of research with demonstrated safety improvements. CRM training has been implemented in operating rooms [198, 199] with a major push towards the use of checklists and team briefings in the OR [184], including initiatives endorsed by the World Health Organization [293]. Another strand of work towards patient safety and operational efficiency improvement has brought about the implementation of Lean management principles from operations science into healthcare [79, 107] and particularly the surgical environment [134]. Such work has demonstrated that Lean Management has positive impact on patient satisfaction, productivity, cost, quality, and efficiency [13, 79]. Recent standards for the design of medical devices and technology have also addressed the issues of safety stemming from systemic factors by mandating extensive requirements gathering and the use of usability and human-factors oriented approaches from software engineering in the development of any device to be used in hospitals (ISO/IEC 62366:2007 [16], ANSI/AAMI-74: 2001 [9], ANSI/AAMI-75:2009 [18], ANSI/AAMI48:1993 [2] and [91, 92]). FMEA, from reliability engineering, has been utilized by some hospitals during process changes and technology integration [21, 73, 277, 292]. Issues of inter-professional communication, relating to power dynamics and safety, have surfaced in the discussions of professional circles [179, 189, 237], but no specific formal standards to address these have been established. Finally, recent efforts from academic environments attempted to bring to the healthcare field the methods from systems engineering – specifically, the stakeholder concerns approach [252, 253].

In summary, attempts have been made to apply some of the approaches from the aviation, reliability engineering, production and manufacturing, software and systems engineering industries (reviewed in Appendix D.1) to the surgical setting. In the next section, the challenges faced by these efforts are discussed. Specifically, challenges are reviewed that have adversely impacted the success and diffusion of improvement initiatives.

6.2.2 Challenges

Despite the numerous efforts to improve communication, coordination, safety and efficiency in the surgical setting and beyond, dramatic diffusion across hospitals, technologies and countries has not been observed. Improvements have been reported in isolated cases, and sometimes follow-up research has identified issues of sustainability of improvements, technology adoption issues alongside positive outcomes, and bias in success stories (see Section 4.5.3 and [98, 148, 160, 176]). Through the research of this study, several challenges to the greater impact of improvement efforts were observed on the macro level of surgical operations:

- Efforts are dispersed and non-systematic. Usually an external consulting group works with a surgical or other hospital unit's management to advise on rapid improvement strategies/programs (as in [79]), without continuous involvement and re-analysis of the state of operations past the initial evaluation, which usually resulted in certain successful metrics.
- Lean management improvements have often been applied on a superficial level of operational changes related to medication stock and operating time efficiency, ignoring the core principles that make Lean work, which require an organizational cultural change where continuous improvement is a value and formal channels of communication between front-line workers and management are established to enable it. (The application of CRM suffers from similar drawbacks as it directly adopts solutions from aviation without considering their evolution in that particular context.)
- There are no communication/coordination standards or active involvement of non-clinical personnel in the establishment of communication practices – there is a lack of multidisciplinary contributions in the determination of communication and coordination practices, which are left at the discretion of the clinical unit.
- Flexibility has been appropriated a high priority, many times overriding adherence to SOPs and frequently resulting in breakdowns and overhead in resolving them. Lack of compliance is pervasive to many procedures, including the use of checklists [176], surgical site marking and performing a "time-out" [148], and CRM procedures in the OR [98]. From the perspective of a

continuous improvement culture, there is a need to address the underlying reasons: Is this a product of perioperative culture? Are the procedures inadequate? Is it both?

- CRM improvement efforts so far have focused on the micro-system level of teamwork within the OR. However, communication and coordination issues span the entire surgical system and, as in aviation, CRM should be applied beyond the single team in the operating room and to the macro system level as well.
- A non-punitive culture of continuous improvement is not the status quo. While in some cases adverse events are brought to light and used to bring on multidisciplinary perspectives to identify proximal and latent factors contributing to breakdowns and to improve patient care (as in [1]), in other cases legislation and politics mandate punishment for any preventable errors [56, 245]. Research across countries and continents shows a high level of defensive medicine practices that come from fear of medical litigation and fear of negative publicity [50]. Punitive legislation promotes the disguise of breakdowns and accidents, the adoption of defensive care practices, and the disabling of any potential for continuous safety improvement.
- Power dynamics, especially between surgeons and nurses, are a major disabler of continuous improvement.
- During improvement initiatives for communication, coordination, safety or efficiency, in-hospital or consultant-lead studies advertise success of programs on a variety of metrics. However, field academic research shows poor performance on similar metrics or on other intervention by-product performances. This is a result of the use of electronic data for fast automated statistical reporting of business and quality metrics utilized in the intervention evaluations by hospitals and consultants – *e.g.* patient throughput, patient visit duration, clinical outcomes, patient satisfaction, and self-report evaluations. These measures neglect to account for important socio-technical dimensions of work - *e.g.* workload, stress, information flow quality, culture, process distance from optimal efficiency, etc. The business metrics also confine analysis to the department/unit neglecting problems at the macro-system level. Field research, mostly coming from academic studies, examines actual behaviors in-context, including macro-level latent factors, but generally is not part of current intervention evaluation processes.

6.2.3 Areas for future work

Given the great number of adverse events and hospital budget considerations, the problem of management of breakdowns and other latent factors endangering safety and undermining efficiency in the perioperative environment needs to be addressed in a more systematic and aggressive fashion. Having identified the major approaches to breakdown management in other industries (in Appendix D.1), and the challenges and disablers to the efforts to implement those approaches in healthcare (in the previous section), several critical areas for future work have emerged.

- **Research.** More research on breakdowns at the macro system level is necessary. The present study expanded the current knowledge in this direction by identifying inter-team breakdowns as primary latent factors for consideration and by revealing how some of the properties of breakdowns statistically determine their consequences. However, this study was only an initial step in the quest to identify and understand macro-level breakdowns. A further look at dysfunctional socio-technical micro-system interactions is necessary in order to address all of the underlying causes.
- **Multidisciplinary approach.** There is a critical need for adoption of a multidisciplinary approach to breakdown management in surgical care units – currently clinical personnel and management with clinical background are the supervisors of breakdown problems and improvement projects. While their input is essential, the contribution of experts with engineering, social science, and human factors perspectives is crucial in addressing systemic latent factors issues. These experts should be involved in the design and evaluation of communication processes and technology in a surgical unit.
- **Systemic approach.** Interventions and technology implementations should be anticipated and evaluated with an outlook on the macro continuum of care, not with a narrow focus on a single micro-system - e.g. the OR – which promotes fragmentation and breakdowns at team interfaces. The involvement of multidisciplinary teams is essential in meeting this requirement.
- **Culture change.** The often punitive and hierarchical culture in surgery is a major disabler to efficient information flow. A balance between flexibility and compliance to procedures and safety is needed. Front-line workers/end-users of processes and technologies should be empowered with formal and direct channels of communication to enable and drive continuous improvement. Most importantly, feedback loops should be formalized so that clinicians can see the outcomes of their potential initiatives to improve the status quo. A long-standing problem with adverse event reporting systems in healthcare is the lack of feedback – when an issue is reported – the reporting party does not usually get invited to contribute to efforts for improvement. Often, the reporting party does not know how and whether the information was used in a productive manner. Even worse, if the issue has seriously affected patient safety, punitive

action may be taken. A formal communication feedback loop is necessary, along with a non-punitive environment so that safety and efficiency are continually improved through the re-design of breakdown contributing mechanisms. The issue of power dynamics between physicians, nurses, administration and management need to be addressed through appropriately designed decision and communication procedures with the goal to enable a safety culture. Only when these conditions are present will techniques such as Lean and CRM truly work.

Cultural change is not an easy task and takes time to evolve and mature. However, aviation is an example of its feasibility – aviation experienced the same types of challenges (*e.g.* power dynamics, micro-system focus, punitive culture) that were overcome through a top-down and systematic approach to training and evaluation facilitated by multidisciplinary inputs. Governmental and corporate endorsement are necessary in promoting a non-punitive culture, pushing towards disabling the forces of power dynamics in patient care, and involving non-clinical experts in all process and safety improvement efforts.

- **Continuous efforts.** Breakdown management requires continuous monitoring of performance post interventions and technology integration, rather than short-term rapid improvement projects. Evaluation metrics should always include both business metrics and socio-technical measures.
- **Flexibility vs. compliance.** The right balance between compliance to procedures and flexibility needs to be determined and potentially standardized in the form of system boundaries for the execution of tasks. Clear system boundaries are necessary to establish productive flexibility vs. flexibility that facilitates inefficiency and safety hazard triggers.
- **No breakdown propagation.** Boundaries should establish disabler checkpoints of patient care when information is missing or incorrect. All other industries reviewed adopt a no propagation policy, recognizing the exponential impact that propagated breakdowns incur. This study showed that propagation is commonplace in perioperative operations and it is the primary communication overhead factor.
- **Prevention vs. avoidance and mitigation.** Greater focus should be appropriated on methods for prevention of communication and coordination breakdowns, rather than on avoidance and mitigation. Given the amount of uncertainty inherent in surgical process operations, avoidance and mitigation techniques are essential for coping with unexpected situations. However, prevention should be priority for recurrent and for preventable breakdowns. The patterns of coordination found in this study, as well as the research literature on the use of workarounds in clinical work, demonstrate a culture with a focus on

avoidance and mitigation of breakdowns.

- **Technology design.** Technology cannot solve the problems that cause breakdowns. First the reasons for breakdowns have to be addressed, and then technology can facilitate the solutions that will prevent, avoid or mitigate breakdowns. Thus, technology has the great potential to improve communication, coordination, safety, and efficiency if designed from a systems engineering perspective and when integrated in a continuous improvement culture. Stakeholder-oriented engineering approaches can greatly enhance the quality and outcome of technology engineering for the surgical environment and should be given further attention in the future.
- **Technology adoption.** Cultural factors, such as *trust*, and a discrepancy in the outcomes from various technology evaluation techniques are the major disablers to accurately identifying and addressing issues of adoption. Future work should focus on the development of accurate predictable user experience (UX) models and on bridging the gap between evaluation approaches. (These ideas were further elaborated on in Section 6.1.4)

Table 28 summarizes the areas of future work required in the management of breakdowns in the perioperative process.

Table 28. Future work for the management of breakdowns.

A need for	*With a focus on*
Research	• macro system level breakdowns • dysfunctional socio-technical system component interactions
Multidisciplinary approach	Experts with engineering, social science, and human factors perspectives should be involved in design and evaluation of communication processes and technology
Systemic approach	All process interventions should anticipate macro-level impact, especially at team/unit interfaces
Culture change	• Non-punitive culture • Continuous improvement driven from the front-line workers • Formal channels of communication, with a closed feedback loop • Procedures to moderate the effects of power dynamics
Continuous efforts	Continuous monitoring rather than rapid-improvement projects
Flexibility vs. compliance	System boundaries to allow for productive flexibility and to prevent inefficiency and safety threatening conditions
No breakdown propagation	System boundaries disabling patient care flow upon missing or incorrect information
Prevention vs. avoidance and mitigation	Greater focus on breakdown prevention
Technology design	• After identifying the reasons for breakdowns, technology can facilitate the solutions • Systems engineering approaches are especially relevant to the issues of inter-team breakdowns • A continuous improvement culture is a precondition to successful integration and long-term adoption
Technology adoption	• development of accurate predictable UX models • research on the discrepancy between self-reported attitudes and observable behaviors

The directions for future work are broad categories independent of particular techniques. While techniques such as CRM and Lean have been applied to the healthcare domain with some success, translation of their application from other fields is not straightforward and requires some important considerations of the differences between the domains [127, 154]. For example, when adopting approaches from the aviation field, it is important to take into account that in the surgical setting the surgeon's life is not threatened during an adverse event. This fact contrasts with the pilot's life in a cockpit situation. Other differences between aviation and surgery range from the level of uncertainty and unpredictability, which is higher for the surgical domain [128], to the hiring process, the initial operating experience, recurrent mandatory training, the management of emergencies, and practice certification requirements [154]. These considerations can have profound implications for the openness to procedure compliance, for decision making, for communication practice, etc. Therefore, an application of CRM or other techniques must be adapted in order to produce optimal results for the surgical setting. When Lean is considered, several value dimensions are relevant in surgical patient care – the clinical, the operational and the patient experience [314]. So far, the majority of accounts of Lean applications to healthcare have looked predominantly at the operational dimension only. As a derivative of reducing the patient's length of stay, these applications have also reported improved patient experience.

Multidisciplinary teams, composed of clinicians and experts in systems engineering, social science, human factors, and operations, are best equipped with the necessary knowledge to determine appropriate process modifications so that procedures and tools would adequately fit the target domain. An example of successful integration of multidisciplinary knowledge into a healthcare domain is the field of Anesthesia where for over thirty years the adoption of systems and human factors perspectives, and recent considerations of reliability engineering concepts and continuous improvement approaches to procedures, has tremendously improved safety [101].

Breakdown management in surgical care can be accomplished with a systematic and well-informed approach. The breakdown detection method, described in the previous chapter, is an essential tool in identifying breakdowns and establishing a baseline for intervention evaluation. Next, breakdowns mechanisms must be identified through a multidisciplinary systemic approach and the process under consideration must be re-designed with the active participation of front-line workers. Clear system boundaries that allow flexibility but also enforce compliance with procedures must be defined. Breakdown propagation must be minimized within the defined system boundaries. The focus of re-design should be on prevention, if possible. A system can often benefit from the advantages of a well designed communication technology. The breakdown detection method should be used to evaluate the outcomes of improvement efforts. However, continuous monitoring and improvement will be key factors in achieving operational efficiency, smooth coordination at team interfaces, and improving safety.

6.3 Chapter summary

The chapter presented a set of guidelines for process and technology (re-)design tailored to the perioperative setting. These guidelines draw on the findings of this research and integrate those findings with the insights from other industries. The guidelines recommend design activities that look beyond tasks and workflows, consider information needs at the macro level, push breakdown disablers away from the day of surgery, anticipate breakdowns not only from a human factors oriented perspective but also from a large-scale coordination perspective, and establish a balance between flexibility and procedure compliance. The guidelines were positioned in the context of the process/technology development lifecycle to produce a coherent system design framework for breakdown management for the surgical setting. The major contribution of the guidelines and framework is the shift in focus during design to latent factors influencing surgical work – healthcare system level processes and breakdowns. By addressing latent factors early in design, the goals of improving safety and efficiency will be attained sooner and at a lower cost. The framework can be applied during early (re-)design stages, but also can be utilized in the context of procedure and software integration over existing hospital processes and implementations, as well as in hospital IT infrastructures design.

The chapter also portrayed some of the challenges to breakdown management in the surgical setting – lack of systematic and multidisciplinary approach to improvement efforts, focus on tools for improvement and neglect for underlying systemic factors such as culture, power dynamics in the OR, etc. The challenges and the knowledge from other domains lead to the conclusion that directions for future work are further research on macro system level breakdowns and on technology adoption issues, a multidisciplinary and systems approach to the detection of breakdowns and to the development of interventional solutions, professional culture changes, continuing efforts at improvement rather than short-lived projects, etc.

7

Conclusion

This chapter summarizes the key findings of this research and discusses critical aspects thereof. In addition, it outlines the theoretical and practical contributions of the book, and discusses some of the limitations of the work. The chapter ends with a discussion of future prospects.

Breakdowns in surgical patient care have been investigated by a number of studies, but the majority confined the scope of analysis to the teamwork frame, while the rest did not examine the deep features of breakdowns. The goal of this research was to analyze breakdowns in the surgical process at a fine level of detail, to reach beyond the unit of a team, and to discover deep features of breakdowns. In this book, a formal systematic study of breakdowns in two OR suites was reported. The scope was set at the perioperative macro-system level, exploring those issues that fluidly move through the surgical process, addressing inter-team coordination, communication cost, and repair strategies. The focus was on the types of breakdowns usually identified as latent factors in adverse events – human errors, coordination breakdowns (including those triggered by unpredictable dynamic conditions) and technical failures. This research applied a mixed methods design. Activity theory, workflow analysis and the systems engineering perspective were employed for the investigation of breakdown factors in a qualitative manner. The micro-systems were modeled and analyzed. Thematic coding and statistical analyses were utilized for quantitative analysis.

In the theoretical domain, the findings were positioned at the intersection of two theoretical models – one of organizational coordination, and the other of cooperation triggered upon breakdowns. A conceptual model of breakdowns in surgical activities was deductively derived. In line with the systems engineering perspective the conceptual model of system behavior reflects a system state as one of *breakdown* or *normal.* The model provides a description of the relationships among breakdown properties examined in this study. Future refinements and further validation of the links are deemed beneficial. Nevertheless, at present the model facilitates an improved understanding of the dependencies of organizational mechanisms and their relationship to breakdowns. Additionally, a model of safety and its relationship to breakdowns was proposed. This model was developed with respect to the findings as well. The safety model is informative not only in understanding the safety implications of breakdowns according to pre-existing communication structures, but also in the design of coordination mechanisms into the surgical process.

In the practical realm, this book offered a breakdown detection method to facilitate the manual and automated detection of breakdowns. Further, guidelines for design and a system design framework were proposed for the design of processes and technologies that prevent existing breakdowns and avoid introducing new ones at integration. The study results suggested that during early design stages as well as during infrastructure design or technology integration, the focus of activity and requirements analysis must be expanded from the user/team unit to the macro-system unit. Technology effects at inter-team interfaces are prime targets of consideration, and barriers should be embedded to prevent breakdowns from downstream propagation in the system process. Finally, coordination requirements with respect to themes, repair structures and tangibility of coordination should be considered in order to provide suitable design solutions.

7.1 Key Findings

The goal of this book was to acquire understanding towards three important questions that will help determine how to improve surgical care coordination through the informed design of processes and technology.

Breakdowns – what are they, really?

This book began the study of breakdowns by deriving breakdown properties and hypotheses from previous qualitative empirical studies and then setting out to explore the relationships between those properties and test the hypotheses with data acquired from real perioperative work in two hospitals. The findings indicated that intra-team micro-system coordination was smooth, while inter-team macro-system level coordination suffered perpetual breakdowns. The sources of these breakdowns were colliding pressures and goals of different teams, maintaining awareness of macro-level plan changes through the alignment of multiple instances of coordinating artifacts, and coordination of tightly coupled actions while in distributed physical spaces.

It was also found that breakdowns originate throughout the surgical macro system and they usually propagate downstream before they are detected and rectified – this was the case in 86% of cases at Hospital_1 and 88% of cases in Hospital_2. As a result, the majority of breakdowns are associated with and affect inter-team coordination. One of the consequences of propagation is that the length of propagation determines the amount of increase in communication cost associated with breakdown repair – the longer the distance from breakdown origin to breakdown detection and repair, the higher the cost. This is probably due to the fact that as they propagate, breakdowns affect the work of a greater number of people. Another reason for this correlation is the increased criticality of process inputs as a patient approaches surgery. Additionally, 68% of breakdown cost is made up of interruptions to the ongoing work of clinicians from various teams. Thus, breakdowns are a major source of interruptions, which has been shown to have significant implications for patient safety.

The breakdown theme was found to relate to the tangibility of the coordination process employed. The breakdown theme predictors were patient information and patient status. The former related to the tangible coordination mechanisms such as paper and electronic artifacts. The vast majority of patient status breakdowns were associated with cultural norms, i.e. the intangible norms and conventions of the local work practice, which supports the idea that cultural norms are predominant in all medical settings [59, 112].

The type of repair strategy employed was determined by a combination of the theme and tangibility associated with a breakdown. Breakdowns related to tangible coordination mechanisms tend to be repaired with information push, while the choice is information pull for breakdowns related to the intangible. As far as breakdown theme is concerned, patient status breakdowns tended to utilize information pull repairs. In Hospital_1, patient information and patient care breakdowns exhibited an information push bias. Although not statistically significant, biases in repair strategy were observed for the other breakdown themes as well.

The study that examined the adoption of the eWhiteboard tool for patient care coordination found that the socio-organizational factor of lack of trust between teams was an enabler of breakdowns and a disabler of successful technology adoption. Even though the eWhiteboard reflected the status of surgical patients correctly, oftentimes clinicians opted to use the phone to verify that the status is indeed accurate. Their comments in-situ revealed that they do not feel confident clinicians from other teams (than their own) had updated the status of patients on the eWhiteboard. This mistrust resulted in a number of phone calls that aimed to verify patient status. Nevertheless, clinicians were highly satisfied with the introduction of the eWhiteboard and perceived it as very useful in their work. The latent factor of lack of trust in the work of other teams was not visible before the introduction of the eWhiteboard as the medium of communication had been the phone – a synchronous medium that allows teams to verify all issues. It is suggested that organizational culture factors should receive greater attention in the future during technology adoption evaluation.

Altogether, the findings reported in this work highlight the need to minimize risk and reduce process waste by addressing breakdowns on a macro-system process level with consideration of coordination mechanisms already in place. The opportunities for breakdown propagation need to be diminished. The implication is that stricter measures are necessary so all necessary inputs at transition points in patient care are in place. Instead of breakdowns being disablers of patient care, breakdown disablers embedded in the system processes are necessary. The properties of breakdowns and their respective repairs need to be exploited in process and system design.

How can breakdowns be detected and measured?

An important insight of this research was that the problem of breakdowns in surgical work lies at macro-system process-level information exchanges. A review of breakdown detection work in other domains proved that a focus on information flow is essential to the detection of problematic information exchanges, *i.e.* breakdowns. It was concluded and proven that breakdown detection in surgical work can be achieved manually or automatically, through a cross-examination of actual information flow between providers of care and expected information flow that is previously modeled. The detection allows to assess the severity with which breakdowns occur, as well as to identify information exchange links that most commonly produce breakdowns. The ability to detect breakdowns provides a meaningful way to design solutions and evaluate improvement interventions.

How can processes and technology be designed to prevent breakdown occurrence?

The relationships found among breakdown and repair properties provide critical knowledge into the specific requirements of coordination that process and technology design should address in an effort to prevent breakdowns. The direct association between properties can be exploited in both technology design and organizational design. Repair efforts can be facilitated with appropriate means of communication. More importantly, the patterns of repair work can inform system design so as to provide clinicians with the types of information that will prevent breakdowns from occurring. A review of the approaches for breakdown prevention in other domains, along with the insights from this research resulted in the following set of design guidelines:

(I) Mind the entire process workflow, not only the problem taskflow.

(II) Consider coordination themes with respect to process. Provide efficient means for repair from breakdowns.

(III) Embed barriers in the system that prevent breakdown propagation, or consider re-engineering the process.

(IV) Mind tangibility – it is important to users.

(V) Consider cultural factors.

(VI) Examine recurrent patterns of coordination.

(VII) Examine recurrent breakdowns, pair them with a solution.

(VIII) Integrate task model, system model and workflow model into a coherent Cooperative Surgical Activity Model.

(IX) Focus on joint activity processes – localization of communication and coordination hotspots.

(X) Represent technology in the task model – localization of human-computer interaction and system-system interaction hotspots.

(XI) Design for safety through breakdowns analysis.

(XII) Either entirely replace a repair/coordination structure, or keep it intact.

Further, detailed breakdowns analysis guidelines were presented. Finally, the guidelines were incorporated into a process/technology design framework that instructs as to the appropriate design activities that each guideline can inform. It is believed that the system design guidelines and framework will have significant impact on the prevention of breakdowns through informing the design of processes and technology of the specific requirements of the perioperative domain.

Through answering the above questions, this book provides a thorough understanding of the main research question posed: *How can we improve surgical care coordination through the informed design of processes and technology that addresses the specific requirements of perioperative work and consequently prevents or mitigates the occurrence of breakdowns?*

7.2 Key contributions

7.2.1 Theoretical relevance

In the theoretical realm, this book makes four contributions that advance the knowledge on breakdowns as latent factors in perioperative work, and consequently in patient safety and operations research.

Mixed methods research design

One of the strengths of this research is the use of both quantitative and qualitative data to gain insight into the problem of breakdowns in surgical care work . This area had previously been studied only with a qualitative approach (Chapter 3). The mixed research design produced a richer understanding of breakdowns than was possible with the qualitative studies in the past. The combination of both methods through exploratory analysis, data coding based on theoretically derived categories, hypothesis testing through statistical means, and survey administration, provided a rich data that allowed for a more thorough exploration of the mechanisms underlying breakdowns, as well as for the identification of the most problematic source of breakdowns – inter-team coordination – through clear numerical evidence.

Understanding of breakdowns

Past research identified the significance of communication and coordination breakdowns to patient safety and technology adoption. In particular, previous work originating from various surgical settings and countries described the occurrence of breakdowns and qualitatively established their relationship to safety. The research presented in this book brought the current understanding of breakdowns to a new level. Breakdowns are now more than a high-level concept, they can be defined formally and systematically according to their properties, lifetime, the associated coordination mechanisms, and the impact they will produce on surgical work (Chapter 4). Specifically, this book presented clear evidence that: breakdowns originate throughout the surgical process; the majority of breakdowns propagate downstream, which determines the amount of increase in communication, interruptions and safety cost associated with their repair; the tangibility of the coordination process relates to the breakdown theme, and both relate to the repair strategy.

This book contributes to the knowledge on breakdowns also with quantitative evidence of the implications of breakdowns in the perioperative process at the macro-system level. In particular, this research demonstrated that the majority of breakdowns, 86% for Hospital_1 and 88% for Hospital_2, propagate through the various micro-systems in the process. In addition, it was found that a minority of breakdowns affects intra-team work, but rather the vast majority of breakdowns – 97% in Hospital_1 and 89% in Hospital_2 – affect macro-system level inter-team work. In the area of technology adoption, this book identified mistrust between teams, *i.e.* at micro-system interfaces, as a disabler to successful technology adoption and perpetrator for continued breakdown occurrence.

The novel and detailed understanding of the deep features of breakdowns and their impact on surgical patient care is an initial step towards the management of breakdowns. It sheds light on the question of why previous efforts at communication and coordination improvement in the OR have not yet eliminated the frequent occurrence of breakdowns – because their focus has been on communication at the micro-system level. This research highlights the need for further work on improving communication and coordination, from a process-oriented perspective.

The findings described above, as well as in Chapter 4, and their implications have been published in scientific conferences and journals [269, 270, 272].

Conceptual model of breakdowns in the surgical process

This book contributes to the existing theory in coordination and organizational research, as well as in patient safety, with a theoretical model that conceptualizes the relationship of coordination properties during normal surgical process operations and breakdown properties under breakdown state operations (Chapter 4 and [270]). Previous research had conceptualized dealing with uncertainties and their impact on coordination in non-clinical organizations. This book investigated the occurrence and impact of breakdowns in surgical operations and developed a model, inspired by previous work, describing the coordination mechanisms and dependencies found particularly in perioperative work. The conceptual model can be useful in the process of detection and analysis of breakdowns, as well as in procedure and technology design.

Conceptual model of safety and breakdowns

In the area of patient safety and design thereof, this book offers a model of safety with respect to the occurrence of breakdowns (Chapter 4). The model conceptualizes the finding that, upon a breakdown, the existence of formal recurrent communication structures for re-coordination influences the potential for safety to be affected, regardless of other organizational factors. The model is informative in the design of both processes and technology for the surgical setting, with the goal of breakdown minimization at integration time.

7.2.2 Practical relevance

The novel and detailed knowledge of breakdowns acquired through the empirical studies was used to lay the foundation for the practical problem of breakdown management through process or technology design. Two major contributions were offered in this domain.

Breakdown detection method

The first step towards the management of breakdowns is the ability to reliably and correctly detect them. Given that the problem of breakdowns in surgical work has not been extensively studied, no formal methods for breakdown detection are available. This book reviewed the breakdown detection approaches from other computational and social sciences concerned with this problem and subsequently developed a breakdown detection method for the perioperative domain (Chapter 5 and [274]). At the core of the method is the modeling of information flow at the macro-system level and matching actual information exchanges to the model. The method integrates the findings of the empirical studies of this research with the approaches from other domains. The model can be used for both manual and automated breakdown detection. Validation was carried out with ROC analysis evaluation over the data collected through the empirical studies in both hospitals. The method exhibited excellent detection performance.

Framework for process/technology design

The second step in the management of breakdowns is the ability to design informed improvement interventions through the (re-)design of processes and technologies. So far, such improvements in surgical patient care were informed solely from efforts in other industries. This book reviewed the relevant approaches to breakdown management in other domains and integrated their wisdom with the newly acquired understanding of breakdowns through this research. The result is a set of guidelines and a design framework, specifically tailored to the requirements of the surgical environment (Chapter 6 and [270, 271, 273]). The guidelines specify how designers of processes and technology should analyze task flows and workflows with an eye on macro-system process level breakdowns. Technology effects at inter-team interfaces are prime targets of consideration. Barriers should be implemented to prevent breakdown propagation but flexibility should be embedded in the process as well. Coordination requirements with respect to themes, repair structures and tangibility of coordination should be considered in order to provide suitable design solutions. The design framework positions the guidelines in the context of the system development lifecycle.

7.3 Limitations

The fact that the two hospitals observed were both situated in the same country and city may have had an impact on the reported results through the effects of professional and organizational culture. However, it should be noted that the surgical process in both hospitals is representative of many North American hospital operations – the same operations are described in Mid-Atlantic [200, 243], North Eastern [246], and other U.S. hospitals [206]. In addition, the findings of this research support those reported by others [243] who also found that in the two hospitals they studied, most breakdowns occurred at group boundaries, i.e. at the inter-team level. Therefore, it is concluded that the settings under consideration in this book are representative of at least North American OR units.

Another limitation is that the distribution of breakdowns in the data by type – among human errors, technical and coordination breakdowns – should only be seen as a good estimate. The figures in this book most probably under-report the actual frequencies of occurrence. This is due to the fact that there was one observer for this study who captured breakdowns one location at a time. However, the number of hours and their distribution across several days was uniform for all point of care locations. Another contributing factor to the under-reported figures is that the human errors breakdown type in particular is not always salient and detectable from an observer's point of reference. This could explain the lack of association found between breakdown type and repair strategy.

Despite the shortcomings, the study reported in this book takes a solid step in the quest to address latent safety risks and organizational efficiency issues through system design. The study achieved an initial understanding of the deep features of breakdowns from a process-oriented systems perspective. This understanding laid the groundwork for a theoretical model of breakdowns in surgical activities, as well as a model of safety and breakdowns, and for the development of a system design approach tailored to perioperative work.

7.4 Future work

This book is one of the first to formally address the problem of breakdowns in the perioperative process at the macro-system process level. As a result, the outcomes of this research provide an understanding of breakdowns that is not complete or mature. Future research should build on the acquired knowledge of this work by further expansion of the breakdown properties set and validation of the relationships among properties of breakdowns and repairs. This will not only enhance the understanding of breakdowns as latent system factors in surgical work, but will also allow for the refinement and strengthening of the proposed design guidelines and system design framework.

A call for future work is also made towards the management of breakdowns, as described in Chapter 6 – through an investment in multi-disciplinary approaches to improvement efforts, a systems approach with focus on the process level and micro-system interfaces, a culture change, continuous efforts at improvement rather than rapid improvement projects, a balance between flexibility and compliance, a focus on breakdown and propagation prevention, and an informed technology design. Most importantly, current efforts at improving communication and information flow in the surgical system need to be re-focused so they include not only a human-centered systems perspective, but also a process-oriented systems view. This research has demonstrated that only when the focus is expanded to the macro-system level, where competing interests and complex interactions among micro-systems and teams are considered, will improvement efforts address the majority of breakdowns occurring in everyday surgical care work and affecting patient safety.

Appendices

Appendix A

A.1 Workflow models

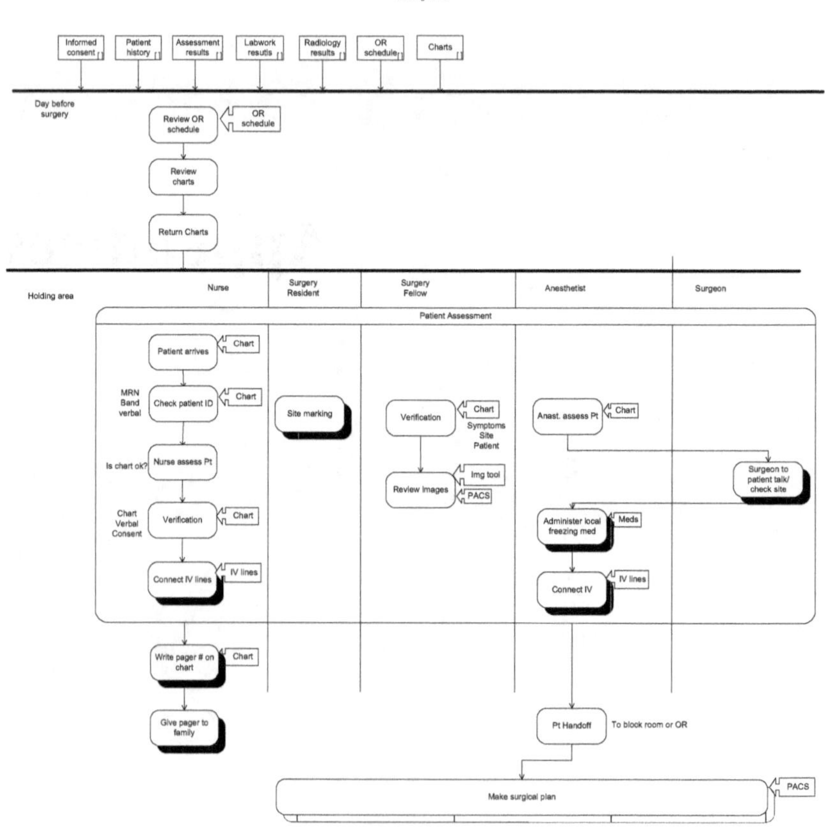

Figure 30: Holding team's workflow.

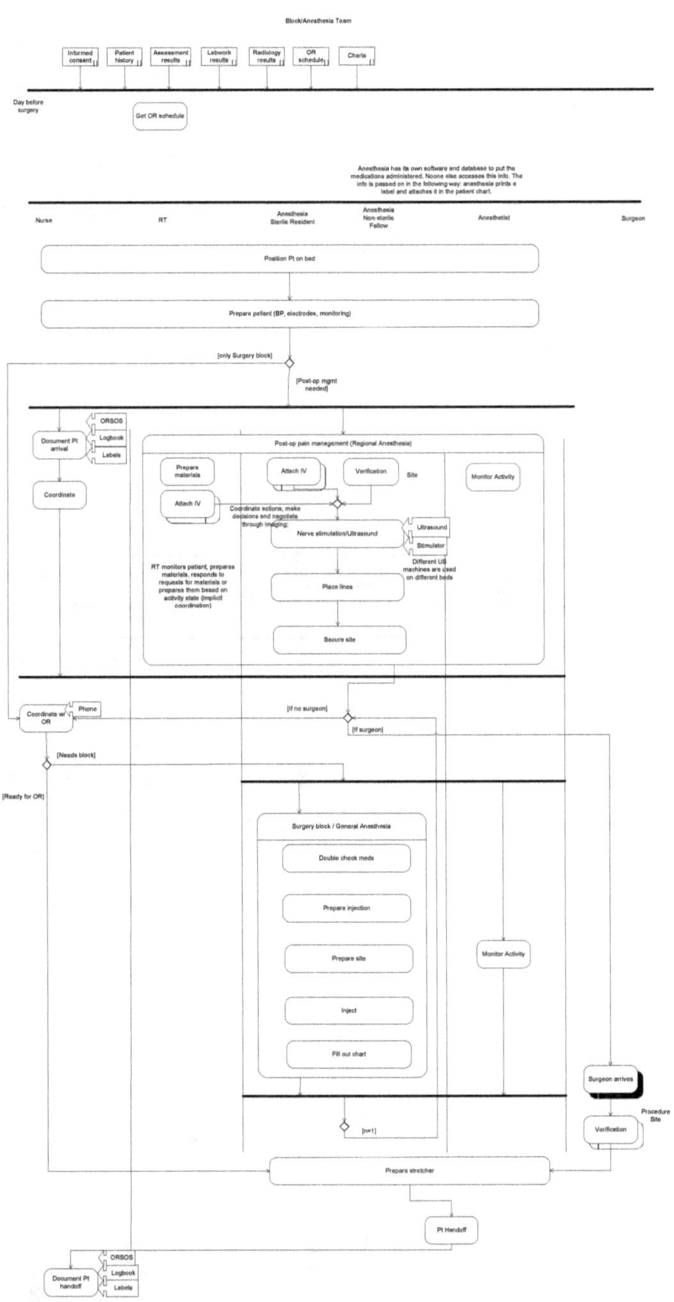

Figure 31: Block/Anesthesia team's workflow.

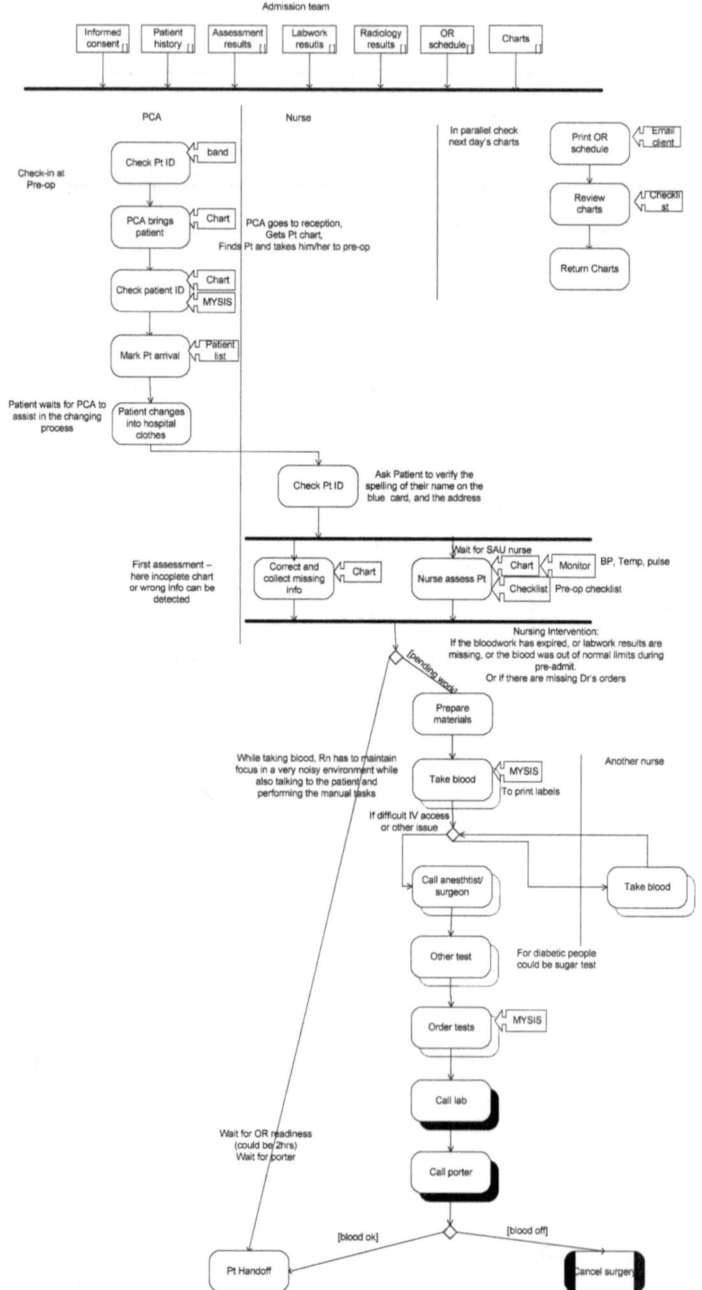

Figure 32: Admission team's workflow.

A.2 Task analysis models

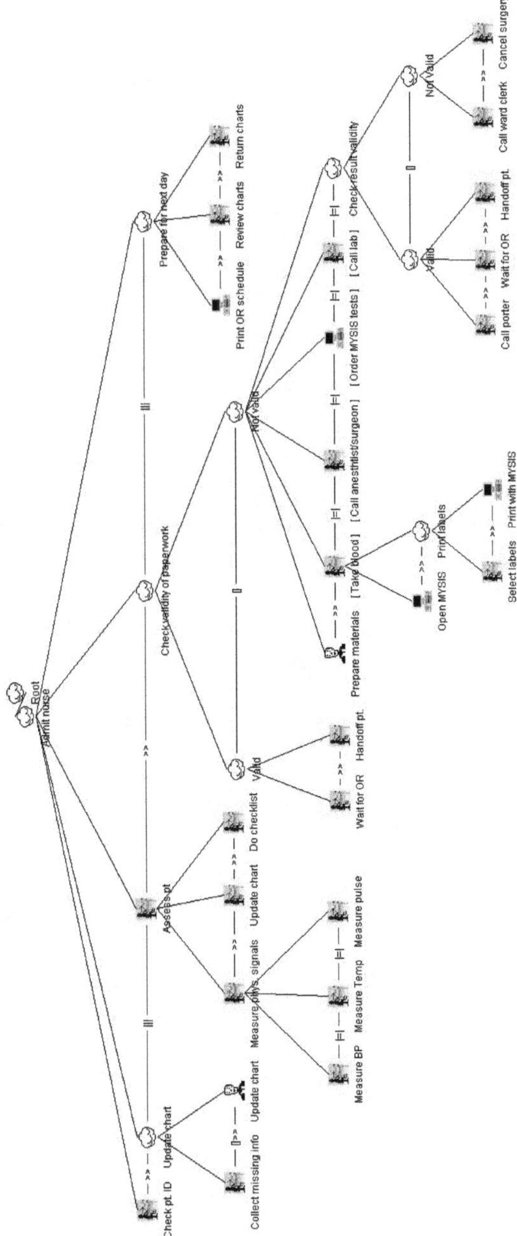

Figure 33: Admission nurse's task model.

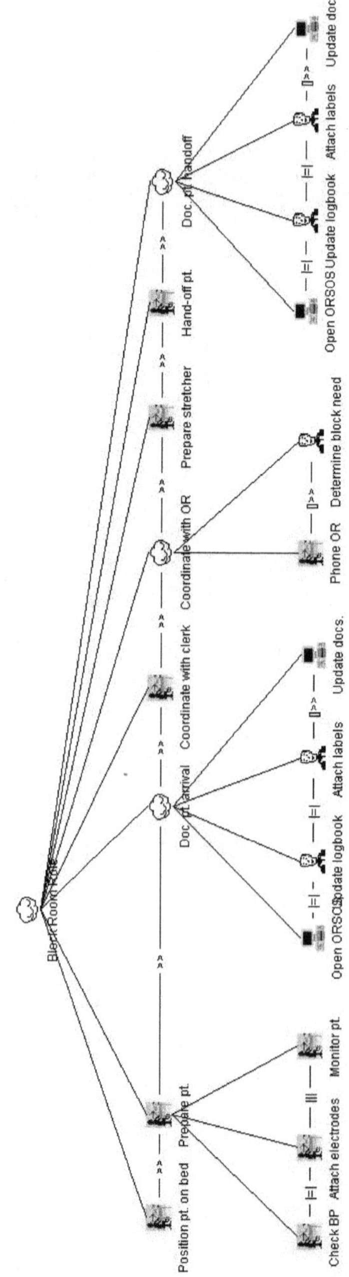

Figure 34: Block/Anesthesia nurse's task model.

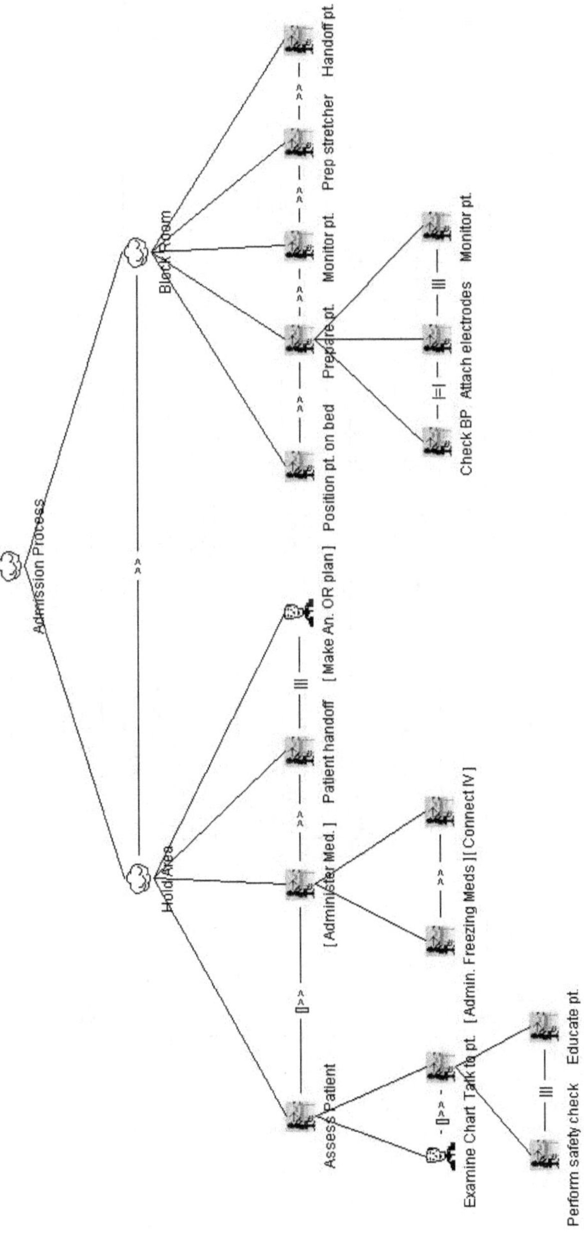

Figure 35: Anesthetist's task model within the block room.

A.3 In-vivo coding scheme

Origin	Target	Event type	Content	Comments	Flag
Receptionist	Receptionist	artifact	OR list	phone	communication breakdown
Patient	Patient	incoming call	EHR	chart	coordination breakdown
PCA	PCA	outgoing call	ORSOS	page	breakdown
Nurse1_Adm	Nurse1_SAU	unsolicited help	GRASP		end breakdown
Nurse2_Adm	Ward Clerk	detect breakdown	slips		interruption
Nurse3_Adm	porter	repair	labels		cancellation
Nurse4_Adm	Nurse2_SAU	explain	pt card		call
OR clerk	Nurse3_SAU	clarification	cklist1		handoff patient
porter	Nurse4_SAU	preparing	cklist2		broadcast
Nurse_Hold	Nurse_HA	message	whiteboard		OR list marking
Anethetist	Anethetist	nod	wristband		trust issue
Surgeon	Ana_Resident	patient response	misplaced sth		Technical failure
Nurse_BlockRm	Ana_Fellow	Criticize	blood		Use error
Family	Surgeon	instruct	cross reference		
Team	Sur_Resident	assessment	lunch		
Blood staff	Sur_Fellow	chat	chart		
Recovery	Nurse_BlockRm	does	schedule		
Imaging staff	RT1	check status	patient care		
Coordinator	RT2	verification	OR readiness		
Nurse5_Adm	Family	double check	patient readiness		
OR	Team	unsolicited info	patient location		
	Imaging staff	ask for help	ID		
	Blood staff	provide help (solicited)	procedure		
	OR staff	monitoring	site		
	None	planning	vitals		
	Other	update pt on actions	patient state		
		question (request info)	patient history		
		reply (provide info)	next patient		
		acknowledge (aha, ok, visible nod)	next day		
		request materials	consent		
		summary on status/plan	equipment		
		coordinate timing of activity	medication		
		instruct	wrong sth		
		offer help	missing sth		
			update pt status		

Figure 36: In-vivo coding scheme.

A.4 Questionnaire

1. How would you rate the pros (advantages) of introducing the whiteboard to your work process?

   (no advantage) 1 2 3 4 5 (improves my work)

2. Can you list some of the advantages

3. How would you rate the cons (DISadvantages) of introducing the whiteboard to your work process?

   (no disadvantage) 1 2 3 4 5 (many disadvantages)

4. Can you list some of the DISadvantages

5. How do you feel when you get a call for a patient whose status on the whiteboard had been accurately updated? (*check one*)

   __ upset __ curious __ doesn't bother me __ angry

6. Why do you think you get such calls? (*check all that apply*)

   __ They don't trust my work, they're checking on me

   __ They don't know how to use the whiteboard

   __ They are making sure everything is ok

   __ Lack of confidence in the whiteboard

   __ Other (specify): ______________________________

   ____

7. How do you feel when you get a call for a patient whose status on the whiteboard is INACCURATE? (*check one*)

   __ guilty __ upset __ curious how it happened __ doesn't bother me

8. Overall, how satisfied are you with the introduction of the whiteboard as a communication tool?

   (not at all) 1 2 3 4 5 (very much)

9. How many years have you worked for the hospital?

   __ 0-5 __ 5-10 __ 10-15 __ 15-20 __ more than 20

Appendix B

B.1 Safety Attitudes Questionnaire (SAQ) and results

Although the SAQ was administered in its entirety, the working conditions dimension has been removed from the table below as it is not relevant to the findings of this research.

The percentage rates for each item represent the means of all positive responses. The percentage rates for each group of items (*e.g.* Teamwork Climate) represent the weighted mean for all respondents' scores within the group of items. The percentage calculation was automatically provided by the SAQ administration tool at http://survey.opensafety.org

The z-score and respective P-value were derived through the two-sample z-test test for proportions.

Table 29. The SAQ and results. $N_{(Hospital\_1)}=17$ and $N_{(Hospital\_2)}=21$.

	hosp1	hosp2	CI	z-score	P (2-tailed)	Significance	Notes
Teamwork Climate	53%	52%	0.95	0.061	0.951		**similarity**
Nurse input is well received in this clinical area.	59%	52%	0.95	0.431	0.666		
it is difficult to speak up if I perceive a problem with patient care.	24%	14%	0.95	0.790	0.430		
Disagreements in this clinical area are resolved appropriately	53%	52%	0.95	0.061	0.951		
I have the support I need from others in this clinical area to care for patients.	65%	67%	0.95	0.130	0.897		
It is easy for personnel here to ask questions when there is something that they do not understand.	76%	67%	0.95	0.608	0.543		
The physicians and nurses here work together as a well-coordinated team.	35%	57%	0.95	1.351	0.177		better at h2
Safety Climate	53%	57%	0.95	0.247	0.805		**similarity**
The culture in this clinical area makes it easy to learn from the errors of others.	56%	52%	0.95	0.246	0.806		
I would feel safe being treated here as a patient.	53%	67%	0.95	0.879	0.380		
Medical errors are handled appropriately in this clinical area.	59%	71%	0.95	0.774	0.439		
I know the proper channels to direct questions regarding patient safety in this clinical area.	59%	81%	0.95	1.488	0.137		
I receive appropriate feedback about my performance.	41%	52%	0.95	0.675	0.499		
In this clinical area, it is difficult to discuss errors.	12%	10%	0.95	0.197	0.844		
I am encouraged by others in this clinical area to report any patient safety concerns I may have.	71%	76%	0.95	0.348	0.728		**difference**
Job Satisfaction	71%	48%	0.95	1.430	0.153		better at h1
I like my job.	88%	67%	0.95	1.516	0.130		better at h1
Working here is like being part of a large family.	53%	48%	0.95	0.307	0.759		
This clinical area is a good place to work.	82%	52%	0.95	1.933	0.053		better at h1, significant at 90CI
I am proud to work in this clinical area.	71%	62%	0.95	0.582	0.560		
Morale in this clinical area is high.	53%	14%	0.95	2.575	0.010	**Significant**	**difference**
Stress Recognition	71%	81%	0.95	0.723	0.470		**similarity**
When my workload becomes excessive my performance is impaired.	76%	71%	0.95	0.346	0.729		
I am less effective at work when fatigued.	82%	90%	0.95	0.716	0.474		
I am more likely to make errors in tense or hostile situations.	76%	95%	0.95	1.704	0.088		better at h2, significant at 90CI
Fatigue impairs my performance during emergency situations (e.g., emergency resuscitation, seizure).	65%	52%	0.95	0.807	0.420		
Unit Management	71%	38%	0.95	2.026	0.043	**Significant**	**difference**
Unit management does not knowingly compromise the safety of patients.	71%	67%	0.95	0.265	0.791		
Unit management supports my daily efforts.	65%	43%	0.95	1.351	0.177		**contributing factor for difference**
I get adequate, timely info about events that might affect my work from unit management.	71%	60%	0.95	0.707	0.480		

B.2 Coded breakdowns data

Hospital	phase	location_num	ID	type	type_num	Theme	theme_num	trigger	trigger_num	tangibility	tangibility_num	scale	scale_num	salience	salience_num	repair	repair_num	cost	d1	d2	d_total
1	1	1	45	dynamic conditions	2	pt care	10	schedule	40		1	inter	2		1	info xfer	3	4	2	2	4
1	1	1	46	coord	1	pt care	10	awareness	4	standard	3	inter and intra	3	implicit	3	info pull	2	2	2	1	3
1	1	1	47	coord	1	pt status	12	awareness	4	standard	3	inter and intra	3		1	info pull	2	2	1	1	2
1	1	1	48	coord	1	pt care	10	awareness	4	standard	3	inter and intra	3		1	info pull	2	5	1	2	3
1	1	1	49	coord	1	pt care	10	materials	16	standard	3	inter and intra	3		1	info pull	2	2	0	1	1
1	1	1	50	dynamic conditions	2	pt care	10	schedule	40		1	inter and intra	3		1	info xfer	3	2	2	4	6
1	1	1	51	coord	1	pt care	10	not enough beds in BR	23	standard	3	intra	4		1	info pull	2	5	0	0	0
1	1	1	52	dynamic conditions	2	pt care	10	schedule	40		1	inter and intra	3		1	info pull	2	3	2	2	4
1	1	1	62	coord	1	pt care	10	missing something	19	standard	3	inter	2	implicit	3	info xfer	3	1	3	2	5
1	1	1	64	coord	1	pt info	11	blue card	6	artifacts	2	inter and intra	3		1	info pull	2	1	1	1	2
1	1	1	65	dynamic conditions	2	pt care	10	pt status	38		1	inter and intra	3		1	info xfer	3	7	0	1	1
1	1	2	16	technical	4	contactability	2	pager	26		1	inter	2	explicit	2	info xfer	3	2	0	1	1
1	1	2	17	coord	1	pt status	12	awareness	4	standard	3	inter	2		1	info pull	2	2	2	1	3
1	1	2	18	technical	4	contactability	2	phone	28		1	inter	2	explicit	2	info xfer	3	2	0	1	1
1	1	2	19	coord	1	pt status	12	awareness	4	standard	3	inter	2		1	info pull	2	2	2	1	3
1	1	2	20	human error	3	slip	4	wrong booking code	46	artifacts	2	inter	2	explicit	2	info pull	2	3	1	0	1
1	1	2	21	coord	1	human factor	4	illegible writing	13	artifacts	2	inter	2	explicit	2	info pull	2	4	1	0	1
1	1	2	22	coord	1	interoperability	15	corss reference number	9	artifacts	2	inter	2	implicit	3	info xfer	3	8	2	2	4
1	1	2	23	coord	1	pt status	12	awareness	4	standard	3	inter	2		1	info pull	2	3	2	1	3
1	1	2	24	coord	1	pt care	10	schedule	40		1	inter and intra	3	implicit	3	info xfer	3	14	0	2	2
1	1	2	25	technical	4	equipment	15	water in OR	44		1		1		1	info xfer	3	3	0	2	2
1	1	2	26	coord	1	pt care	10	schedule	40		1	inter	2	implicit	3		1	0	1	0	1
1	1	2	27	coord	1	contactability	2	ask clerk to contact surg	3	standard	3	inter	2	implicit	3	info xfer	3	3	1	1	2
1	1	2	27b	coord	1	pt info	11	prep work	29	artifacts	2	inter	2	implicit	3	info xfer	3	3	2	3	5
1	1	2	28	dynamic conditions	2	contactability	2	nurse is late for work	24		1	inter	2		1	info xfer	3	9	1	1	2
1	1	2	29	coord	1	pt care	10	pt needs wheelchair, po	37	standard	3	inter	2		1	info xfer	3	2	1	1	2
1	1	2	30	dynamic conditions	2	reliability	10	snowstorm, clerk is late	41	standard	3	inter	2	implicit	3	postitive coordinat	1	4	1	4	5
1	1	2	31	coord	1	pt care	10	materials	16	standard	3	inter and intra	3	implicit	3	info pull	2	32	2	2	4
1	1	2	32	dynamic conditions	2	pt care	10	schedule	40		1	inter and intra	3	implicit	3	info xfer	3	9	2	4	6
1	1	2	33	dynamic conditions	2	pt care	10	schedule	40		1	inter and intra	3	implicit	3	info xfer	3	20	2	4	6
1	1	2	34	dynamic conditions	2	pt status	12	awareness	4		1	inter	2	implicit	3	info pull	2	5	3	2	5
1	1	3	35	coord	1	pt info	11	prep work	29	artifacts	2	inter	2	implicit	3	info xfer	3	2	1	2	3
1	1	3	36	dynamic conditions	2	pt care	10	schedule	40		1	inter and intra	3	implicit	3	info pull	2	3	2	4	6
1	1	3	37	coord	1	pt care	10	pt transfer	39	standard and a	4	inter	2	implicit	3	info xfer	3	2	1	1	2
1	1	3	38	human error	3	lapse	4	pt info	35	artifacts	2	inter	2	implicit	3	info pull	2	1	0	0	0
1	1	3	39	coord	1	contactability	2	noone to answer phone	22		1	inter	2	explicit	2		1	####	####	####	#NULL!
1	1	3	40	coord	1	pt care	10	schedule	40		1	inter and intra	3	implicit	3	info pull	2	2	2	4	6
1	1	3	41	coord	1	pt status	12	awareness	4	standard	3	inter	2	implicit	3	info pull	2	1	2	2	4
1	1	3	42	technical	4	contactability	2	trying to contact OR	43	standard	3	inter	2	explicit	2		1	####	1	2	3
1	1	3	43	coord	1	pt status	12	awareness	4	standard	3	inter	2	implicit	3	info pull	2	1	1	0	1
1	1	3	44	coord	1	pt care	10	awareness	4	standard	3	inter	2		1		1	####	####	####	#NULL!
1	1	3	61	coord	1	pt care	10	prep work	29	standard	3	inter	2	implicit	3	info xfer	3	1	2	3	5
1	1	4	1	coord	1	pt info	11	prep work	29	artifacts	2	inter	2	implicit	3	info xfer	3	6	4	4	8
1	1	4	2	coord	1	pt info	11	prep work	29	artifacts	2	inter	2	implicit	3	info xfer	3	10	4	2	6
1	1	4	2a	human error	3	slip	4	wrong call back number	47		1	inter	2		1	info xfer	3	2	0	1	1
1	1	4	3	coord	1	pt care	10	meds	18	standard	3	inter	2	implicit	3	info xfer	3	3	1	1	2
1	1	4	4	dynamic conditions	2	pt care	10	schedule	40		1	inter and intra	3	implicit	3	info xfer	3	10	2	4	6
1	1	4	5	coord	1	pt info	11	prep work	29	artifacts	2	inter	2	implicit	3	info xfer	3	5	3	2	5
1	1	4	6	coord	1	human factor	4	lapse	15	artifacts	2	inter	2	explicit	2	info pull	2	2	3	3	6
1	1	4	7	coord	1	pt care	10	prep work	29	artifacts	2	inter	2	implicit	3	info pull	2	8	4	2	6
1	1	4	8	coord	1	pt care	10	pt transfer	39	standard	3	inter	2	implicit	3	wait	1	0	1	1	2
1	1	4	9	coord	1	pt care	10	blood	5	standard	3	inter	2	implicit	3	info pull	2	7	2	2	4
1	1	4	9a	dynamic conditions	2	pt care	10	schedule	40		1	inter and intra	3	implicit	3	info xfer	3	5	2	4	6
1	1	4	10	dynamic conditions	2	pt care	10	schedule	40		1		1		1	info xfer	3	4	2	2	4
1	1	4	11	coord	1	pt care	10	blood	5	standard	3	inter and intra	3	implicit	3	info xfer	3	3	2	2	4
1	1	4	12	coord	1	pt care	10	schedule	40		1	inter and intra	3	implicit	3	info pull	2	2	2	2	4
1	1	4	13	dynamic conditions	2	pt care	10	schedule	40		1	inter and intra	3	implicit	3	info xfer	3	3	2	4	6
1	1	4	14	coord	1	pt care	10	pt destination	34	artifacts	2	inter	2	implicit	3	info xfer	3	2	1	1	2
1	1	4	15	coord	1	pt info	11	prep work	29	artifacts	2	inter	2	implicit	3	info xfer	3	3	4	2	6
1	1	4	53	coord	1	pt care	10	labelling	14	artifacts	2	inter and intra	3		1	info pull	2	1	0	0	0
1	1	4	54	technical	4	pt care	10	labelling	14	artifacts	2	inter and intra	3		1	info xfer	3	3	1	0	1
1	1	4	55	coord	1	pt info	11	prep work	29	artifacts	2	inter and intra	3		1	info pull	2	4	3	4	7
1	1	4	56	dynamic conditions	2	pt info	11	pt changed address	32	artifacts	2		1		1		1	2	2	0	2

Hospital	phase	location_num	ID	type	type_num	Theme	theme_num	trigger	trigger_num	tangibility	tangibility_num	scale	scale_num	salience	salience_num	repair	repair_num	cost	d1	d2	d_total
1	2	2	121	coord	1	pt status	12	awareness	4	standard	3	inter	2		1	info pull	2	1	2	0	2
1	2	2	122	dynamic conditions	2	pt care	10	schedule	40		1	inter and intra	3		1	info xfer	3	17	2	4	6
1	2	2	123	dynamic conditions	2	pt care	10	pt destination	34		1	inter and intra	3		1	info xfer	3	3	1	0	1
1	2	2	124	coord	1	pt status	12	trust	42	standard	3	inter	2		1	info pull	2	1	1	0	1
1	2	2	125	coord	1	pt status	12	trust	42	standard	3	inter	2		1	info pull	2	1	1	0	1
1	2	2	126	coord	1	pt status	12	trust	42	standard	3	inter	2		1	info pull	2	1	1	0	1
1	2	2	127	coord	1	pt care	10	schedule	40	artifacts	2	inter and intra	3		1	info xfer	3	6	2	4	6
1	2	2	128	dynamic conditions	2	pt care	10	schedule	40		1	inter and intra	3		1	info xfer	3	6	2	4	6
1	2	2	129	coord	1	pt status	12	trust	42	standard	3	inter	2		1	info pull	2	1	1	0	1
1	2	2	130	dynamic conditions	2	pt care	10	patient	27		1	inter and intra	3		1	info xfer	3	2	1	1	2
1	2	3	131	coord	1	pt care	10	blue card	6	artifacts	2	inter and intra	3		1	info xfer	3	2	0	1	1
1	2	3	132	human error	3	mistake	4	pt transfer	39	standard	3	inter	2		1		1	1	0	0	0
1	2	3	133	dynamic conditions	2	pt care	10	patient	27		1	inter and intra	3		1	info xfer	3	12	####	1	#NULL!
1	2	3	134	human error	3	lapse	4	pt transfer	39	artifacts	2	inter	2		1		1	0	0	0	0
1	2	3	135	coord	1	pt care	10	prep work	29	artifacts	2		1		1		1	1	4	1	5
1	2	3	136	technical	4	contactability	2	pager	26		1	inter	2		1		1	1	1	0	1
1	2	3	137	dynamic conditions	2	pt care	10	schedule	40		1	inter and intra	3		1	info pull	2	2	2	0	2
1	2	3	138	coord	1	pt care	10	prep work	29	artifacts	2	inter	2		1	info xfer	3	2	0	2	2
1	2	3	139	coord	1	contactability	2	noone to answer phone	22		1	inter	2		1		1	####	####	####	#NULL!
1	2	3	140	coord	1	pt care	10	prep work	29	artifacts	2	inter	2		1	info xfer	3	2	0	2	2
1	2	3	141	dynamic conditions	2	pt care	10	schedule	40		1	inter and intra	3		1	info xfer and pull	4	10	2	0	2
1	2	3	142	coord	1	pt care	10	blood	5	standard	3	inter	2		1	info xfer and pull	4	4	2	0	2
1	2	3	143	dynamic conditions	2	pt care	10	schedule	40		1	inter and intra	3		1	info xfer	3	4	1	1	2
1	2	3	144	coord	1	pt status	12	trust	42	standard	3	inter	2		1	info pull	2	1	1	0	1
1	2	3	145	coord	1	pt status	12	pt transfer	39	standard	3	inter	2		1	info pull	2	1	1	0	1
1	2	3	146	coord	1	pt care	10	pt marking	36	standard	3	inter	2		1		1	1	1	0	1
1	2	3	147	coord	1	pt care	10	trust	42	standard	3	inter	2		1		1	1	1	0	1
1	2	3	148	coord	1	pt status	12	pt transfer	39	standard	3	inter	2		1	info pull	2	1	1	0	1
1	2	3	149	human error	3	slip	4	whiteboard	45	artifacts	2	inter	2		1		1	1	0	0	0
1	2	3	150a	coord	1	pt care	10	blue card	6	artifacts	2	inter and intra	3		1	info pull	2	2	1	1	2
1	2	3	150b	coord	1	pt care	10	trust	42	standard	3	inter	2		1	info xfer	3	2	1	1	2
1	2	3	151a	coord	1	pt care	10	arm band	2	artifacts	2	inter	2		1	info xfer and pull	4	3	2	2	4
1	2	3	151b	coord	1	pt care	10	trust	42	standard	3	inter	2		1	info xfer	3	1	2	2	4
1	2	3	152	dynamic conditions	2	pt care	10	patient	27		1	inter and intra	3		1		1	1	####	0	#NULL!
1	2	3	153	coord	1	pt care	10	blood	5		1	inter	2		1	info pull	2	4	2	2	4
1	2	3	154	coord	1	pt care	10	prep work	29	standard	3	inter and intra	3		1	info xfer	3	3	5	1	6
1	2	3	155	human error	3	lapse	4	pt coord	33	artifacts	2	inter	2		1	info pull	2	1	0	0	0
1	2	3	156	coord	1	contactability	2	pt cant reach dr	31		1		1		1	info xfer	3	####	####	####	#NULL!
1	2	3	157	technical	4	equipment	15	monitor	20		1	intra	4		1	info xfer	3	2	0	1	1
1	2	3	158	coord	1	pt care	10	prep work	29	artifacts	2		1		1	info xfer	3	3	2	2	4
1	2	4	1	coord	1	pt info	11	prep work	29	standard	3	inter	2	implicit	3	info xfer	3	9	3	2	5
1	2	4	2	dynamic conditions	2	pt care	10	pt coord	33	standard	3	inter and intra	3	implicit	3	info xfer	3	1	1	1	2
1	2	4	3	coord	1	pt info	11	prep work	29	artifacts	2	inter	2	implicit	3	info xfer	3	2	4	2	6
1	2	4	4	coord	1	pt status	12	awareness	4	standard	3	inter and intra	3	implicit	3	info pull	2	2	1	1	2
1	2	4	5	human error	3	human factor	4	prep work	29	artifacts	2	inter	2	explicit	2	info xfer	3	4	4	2	6
1	2	4	6	coord	1	pt info	11	prep work	29	standard	3	inter	2	implicit	3	info xfer	3	5	3	2	5
1	2	4	7	coord	1	pt status	12	trust	42	standard	3	inter	2	implicit	3	info pull	2	4	1	0	1
1	2	4	8	coord	1	pt status	12	trust	42	standard	3	inter	2	explicit	2	info pull	2	1	1	0	1
1	2	4	9	coord	1	pt info	11	prep work	29	artifacts	2	inter	2	explicit	2	info xfer	3	2	3	2	5
1	2	4	10	coord	1	pt status	12	trust	42	standard	3	inter	2		1	info pull	2	2	1	0	1
1	2	4	11	coord	1	pt status	12	trust	42	standard	3	inter	2		1	info pull	2	2	1	0	1
1	2	4	12	coord	1	pt status	12	trust	42	standard	3	inter	2		1		1	2	1	0	1
1	2	4	13	coord	1	pt care	10		1	standard	3	inter	2	implicit	3	info pull	2	1	0	1	1
1	2	4	14	coord	1	pt info	11	prep work	29	artifacts	2	inter and intra	3		1	info xfer	3	4	3	4	7
1	2	4	15	coord	1	pt status	12	trust	42	standard	3	inter	2		1	info pull	2	1	1	0	1
1	2	4	16	coord	1	pt status	12	trust	42	standard	3	inter	2		1	info pull	2	1	2	0	2
1	2	4	17	human error	3	lapse	4	did not see wrong input	11	artifacts	2	inter	2		1		1	1	1	1	2
1	2	4	18	coord	1	pt status	12	trust	42	standard	3	inter	2		1	info pull	2	1	1	0	1
1	2	4	19	human error	3	slip	4	whiteboard	45	artifacts	2	inter	2		1		1	1	0	1	1
1	2	4	19a	human error	3	slip	4	whiteboard	45	artifacts	2	inter and intra	3		1	info xfer	3	2	0	1	1
1	2	4	19b	coord	1	pt status	12	prev error	30	artifacts	2	inter	2		1		1	1	0	0	0
1	2	4	20	coord	1	pt status	12	trust	42	standard	3	inter	2		1	info pull	2	1	1	0	1
1	2	4	21	coord	1	pt info	11	prep work	29	standard	3	inter and intra	3	implicit	3	info xfer	3	1	4	2	6

Hospital	phase	location_num	ID	type	type_num	Theme	theme_num	trigger	trigger_num	tangibility	tangibility_num	scale	scale_num	salience	salience_num	repair	repair_num	cost	d1	d2	d_total
1	2	4	22	coord	1	pt info	11	prep work	29	standard	3		1		1	info xfer	3	3	4	2	6
1	2	4	23	human error	3	pt info	11	lapse	15	artifacts	2	inter and intra	3		1	info pull	2	2	3	1	4
1	2	4	24	coord	1	pt info	11	prep work	29	artifacts	2	inter	2		1	info xfer	3	5	4	2	6
1	2	4	25	coord	1	pt status	12	trust	42	standard	3	inter	2		1	info pull	2	1	1	0	1
1	2	4	26	technical	4	medium	15	whiteboard	45	artifacts	2	inter and intra	3		1	info xfer	3	1	0	1	1
1	2	4	27	coord	1	pt care	10	prep work	29	artifacts	2	inter	2		1	info xfer	3	6	4	2	6
1	2	4	28	dynamic conditions	2	pt care	10	patient	27		1	inter and intra	3		1	info xfer	3	7	####	2	#NULL!
1	2	4	29	human error	3	slip	4	whiteboard	45	artifacts	2	inter	2		1		1	1	0	0	0
1	2	4	30	dynamic conditions	2	pt care	10	patient	27		1	inter and intra	3		1	info xfer	3	12	####	2	#NULL!
1	2	4	31	coord	1	pt care	10	patient	27	artifacts	2	inter	2		1	info xfer	3	8	3	4	7
1	2	4	32	coord	1	pt info	11	prep work	29	artifacts	2	inter	2		1	info xfer	3	9	4	2	6
1	2	4	33	coord	1	pt info	11	prep work	29	artifacts	2	inter	2		1	info xfer	3	3	4	2	6
1	2	4	34	human error	3	lapse	4	whiteboard	45	artifacts	2	inter	2		1		1	1	0	0	0
1	2	4	35	dynamic conditions	2	pt status	12	trust	42	standard	3	inter	2		1	info pull	2	6	1	0	1
1	2	4	36	dynamic conditions	2	pt care	10	patient	27		1	inter and intra	3		1	info pull	2	5	####	2	#NULL!
1	2	4	37	coord	1	pt info	11	prep work	29	artifacts	2	inter	2		1	info xfer	3	4	4	2	6
1	2	4	38	coord	1	pt care	10	pt transfer	39	artifacts	2	inter	2		1		1	2	####	1	#NULL!
1	2	4	39	human error	3	lapse	4	whiteboard	45	artifacts	2	inter	2		1		1	1	1	0	1
1	2	4	40	human error	3	slip	4	whiteboard	45	artifacts	2	inter	2		1		1	1	0	0	0
1	2	4	41	dynamic conditions	2	pt status	12	trust	42	standard	3	inter	2		1	info pull	2	1	1	0	1
1	2	4	42	dynamic conditions	2	pt care	10	schedule	40		1	inter and intra	3		1		1	2	2	1	3
1	2	4	43	coord	1	pt info	11	prep work	29	artifacts	2	inter and intra	3		1	info pull	4	1	1	0	1
1	2	4	44	coord	1	pt info	11	prep work	29	artifacts	2	inter and intra	3		1	info xfer	3	5	3	2	5
1	2	4	45	technical	4	equipment	15	device	10		1	intra	4		1	info xfer and pull	2	6	0	1	1
1	2	4	46	technical	4	info sys	15	mysis	21	artifacts	2	inter and intra	3		1	info pull	2	4	2	2	4
1	2	4	47	coord	1	pt care	10	blue card	6	artifacts	2	inter	2		1	info pull	2	6	2	1	3
1	2	4	48	coord	1	pt status	12	trust	42	standard	3	inter	2		1	info pull	2	1	1	0	1
1	2	4	49	coord	1	pt status	12	trust	42	standard	3	inter	2		1	info pull	2	1	1	0	1
1	2	4	50	coord	1	pt care	10	prep work	29	artifacts	2	inter	2		1	info pull	2	2	2	2	4
1	2	4	51	coord	1	pt care	10	schedule	40		1	inter	2		1	info xfer	3	11	4	3	7
1	2	4	52	coord	1	human factor	4	med order	17		1	inter	2		1	info pull	2	1	4	0	4
1	2	4	53	coord	1	pt care	10	pt transfer	39	standard	3	inter	2		1	info pull	2	3	1	1	2
1	2	4	54	coord	1	pt status	12	trust	42	standard	3	inter	2		1	info pull	2	1	1	0	1
1	2	4	55	coord	1	pt care	10	pt transfer	39	standard	3	inter	2		1		1	1	1	0	1
1	2	4	56	coord	1	pt care	10	schedule	40		1	inter	2		1	info xfer	3	6	2	4	6
1	2	4	57	dynamic conditions	2	pt care	10	schedule	40		1	inter and intra	3		1	info xfer	3	3	2	2	4
1	2	4	58	dynamic conditions	2	pt care	10	schedule	40		1	inter and intra	3		1	info xfer	3	3	2	2	4
1	2	4	59	dynamic conditions	2	pt care	10	schedule	40		1	inter and intra	3		1	info xfer	3	2	2	2	4
1	2	4	60	dynamic conditions	2	pt care	10	patient	27		1	inter and intra	3		1	info xfer	3	4	####	2	#NULL!
1	2	4	61	coord	1	pt info	11	prep work	29	artifacts	2	inter	2		1	info xfer	3	3	4	2	6
1	2	4	61a	coord	1	pt info	11	prep work	29	artifacts	2	inter	2		1	info xfer	3	10	4	2	6
1	2	4	62	dynamic conditions	2	pt care	10	patient	27		1	inter and intra	3		1	info xfer	3	5	####	2	#NULL!
1	2	4	63	coord	1	pt status	12	trust	42	standard	3	inter	2		1	info pull	2	1	1	0	1
1	2	4	64	human error	3	human factor	4	prep work	29		1	inter and intra	3		1	info xfer	3	3	4	2	6
1	2	4	65	human error	3	mistake	4	pt transfer	39		1	inter	2		1		1	3	0	1	1
2	3	2	65	human error	3	pt info	11	arm band	2	artifacts	2	inter	2		1		1	####	####	####	#NULL!
2	3	2	66	coord	1	contactability	2	noone to answer phone	22		1	inter	2		1		1	####	####	####	#NULL!
2	3	2	67	dynamic conditions	2	pt care	10	schedule	40	standard	3		1		1		1	####	####	####	#NULL!
2	3	2	.	coord	1	pt care	10	schedule	40	standard	3	inter	2		1		1	1	1	0	1
2	3	2	.	coord	1	pt care	10	trust	42	standard	3	inter	2		1	info pull	2	2	1	0	1
2	3	2	69	coord	1	contactability	2	noone to answer phone	22		1	inter	2		1	info pull	2	6	2	2	3
2	3	2	70	dynamic conditions	2	pt care	10	schedule	40		1	inter and intra	3		1	info pull	2	6	1	1	2
2	3	2	71	dynamic conditions	2	pt care	10	schedule	40		1	inter and intra	3		1	info xfer	3	2	1	1	2
2	3	2	72	dynamic conditions	2	pt care	10	schedule	40	standard	3	inter	2		1	info xfer	3	####	####	####	#NULL!
2	3	2	73	dynamic conditions	2	pt care	10	schedule	40		1	inter and intra	3		1	info xfer	3	4	####	####	#NULL!
2	3	2	74	dynamic conditions	2	pt care	10	schedule	40		1	inter and intra	3		1		1	2	0	1	1
2	3	2	75	dynamic conditions	2	pt care	10	schedule	40	standard	3		1		1	info xfer and pull	4	1	1	1	2
2	3	2	76	dynamic conditions	2	pt care	10	patient	27	standard	3	intra	4		1	info pull	2	2	0	0	0
2	3	2	77	dynamic conditions	2	pt care	10	schedule	40		1		1		1	info pull	2	3	2	1	3
2	3	2	78	coord	1	pt status	12	pt transfer	39	standard	3	inter and intra	3		1	info pull	2	3	1	1	2
2	3	2	79	dynamic conditions	2	pt care	10	schedule	40		1	inter and intra	3		1	info xfer and pull	4	5	2	1	3
2	3	2	80	coord	1	pt care	10	pt transfer	39	artifacts	2		1		1		1	1	1	0	1
2	3	2	81	dynamic conditions	2	pt care	10	schedule	40		1	inter and intra	3		1	info pull	2	10	1	1	2

Hospital	phase	location_num	ID	type	type_num	Theme	theme_num	trigger	trigger_num	tangibility	tangibility_num	scale	scale_num	salience	salience_num	repair	repair_num	cost	d1	d2	d_total
2	3	2	82	dynamic conditions	2	pt care	10	schedule	40		1		1		1	info pull	2	3	1	1	2
2	3	2	83	coord	1	pt care	10	schedule	40		1	intra	4		1		1	9	3	0	3
2	3	2	84	coord	1	pt status	12	awareness	4		1	inter	2		1	info xfer and pull	4	7	####	####	#NULL!
2	3	2	85	dynamic conditions	2	pt care	10	schedule	40		1		1		1	info pull	2	1	1	0	1
2	3	2	86	dynamic conditions	2	pt care	10	schedule	40		1		1		1	info pull	2	1	1	0	1
2	3	2	87	dynamic conditions	2	pt care	10	schedule	40		1		1		1	info xfer and pull	4	10	1	1	2
2	3	2	88	dynamic conditions	2	pt care	10	schedule	40		1	inter	2		1	info xfer	3	1	0	1	1
2	3	2	89	technical	4	medium	15	phone	28		1	inter	2		1	info xfer	3	6	1	2	3
2	3	2	90	dynamic conditions	2	pt care	10	schedule	40		1	inter and intra	3		1	info xfer	3	1	1	1	2
2	3	2	91	dynamic conditions	2	pt care	10	schedule	40		1	inter	2		1	info xfer and pull	4	10	####	####	#NULL!
2	3	2	92	coord	1	pt status	12	awareness	4	standard	3	inter	2		1	info pull	2	1	1	1	2
2	3	2	93	dynamic conditions	2	pt care	10	schedule	40	standard	3	inter and intra	3		1		1	18	2	1	3
2	3	2	94	dynamic conditions	2	pt care	10	schedule	40		1		1		1	info pull	2	1	1	0	1
2	3	2	95	dynamic conditions	2	pt care	10	schedule	40	standard	3	inter	2		1	info pull	2	2	0	1	1
2	3	2	96	coord	1	pt status	12	awareness	4	standard	3	inter	2		1		1	1	1	0	1
2	3	2	97	coord	1	pt care	10	schedule	40		1		1		1		1	8	1	1	2
2	3	2	98	coord	1	pt status	12	awareness	4	standard	3	inter	2		1	info pull	2	5	1	2	3
2	3	2	99	coord	1	pt care	10	schedule	40	artifacts	2	inter and intra	3		1	info pull	2	2	1	1	2
2	3	2	100	coord	1	pt care	10	pt status	38	standard	3	inter and intra	3		1	info xfer	3	2	2	2	4
2	3	2	101	dynamic conditions	2	pt care	10	patient	27		1	inter and intra	3		1	info xfer	3	2	####	1	#NULL!
2	3	2	102	dynamic conditions	2	pt care	10	schedule	40		1	inter and intra	3		1	info xfer	3	34	2	3	5
2	3	2	.	coord	1	pt care	10	prep work	29	standard	3	inter and intra	3		1	info xfer	3	24	1	3	4
2	3	2	.	coord	1	pt status	12	awareness	4	standard	3	inter	2		1	info pull	2	3	1	1	2
2	3	2	.	coord	1	contactability	2	noone to answer phone	22	standard	3	inter	2		1	info xfer	3	3	0	1	1
2	3	2	103	coord	1	pt care	10	z_staffing	48	standard	3	inter and intra	3		1	info xfer	3	5	0	2	2
2	3	2	104	technical	4	medium	15	phone	28		1	inter and intra	3		1	info xfer	3	2	0	2	2
2	3	2	105	human error	3	slip	4	phone	28		1		1		1		1	2	1	0	1
2	3	2	106	dynamic conditions	2	pt care	10	schedule	40	standard	3	inter and intra	3		1	info xfer and pull	4	6	1	3	4
2	3	2	107	coord	1	pt care	10	device	10		1		1		1	info xfer and pull	4	4	2	0	2
2	3	3	108	coord	1	pt care	10	prep work	29	artifacts	2	inter and intra	3		1	info xfer	3	3	2	1	3
2	3	3	109	coord	1	pt status	12	awareness	4	standard	3	inter and intra	3		1	info pull	2	14	0	0	0
2	3	3	110	dynamic conditions	2	pt care	10	schedule	40		1	inter and intra	3		1	info xfer	3	5	2	1	3
2	3	3	111	dynamic conditions	2	pt care	10	patient	27		1	inter and intra	3		1	info xfer	3	2	2	1	3
2	3	3	112	dynamic conditions	2	pt care	10	schedule	40		1	inter and intra	3		1	info xfer and pull	4	7	1	2	3
2	3	3	113	coord	1	contactability	2	noone to answer phone	22		1	inter	2		1		1	1	####	####	#NULL!
2	3	3	114	dynamic conditions	2	pt care	10	schedule	40		1	inter and intra	3		1	info pull	2	2	1	1	2
2	3	3	115	coord	1	pt status	12	pt transfer	39	standard	3	inter	2		1	info pull	2	2	1	1	2
2	3	3	116	coord	1	contactability	2	noone to answer phone	22		1	inter	2		1		1	1	####	####	#NULL!
2	3	3	117	coord	1	pt info	11	prep work	29	artifacts	2	inter	2		1	info xfer	3	3	3	1	4
2	3	3	118	coord	1	pt info	11	prep work	29	artifacts	2	inter	2		1	info xfer	3	2	3	1	4
2	3	3	119	dynamic conditions	2	pt care	10	patient	27		1	inter and intra	3		1	info xfer	3	1	####	####	#NULL!
2	3	3	.	coord	1	pt care	10	schedule	40	artifacts	2	inter	2		1	info pull	2	4	1	1	2
2	3	3	.	coord	1	pt info	11	prep work	29	artifacts	2	inter	2		1	info xfer	3	2	1	1	2
2	3	3	121	coord	1	pt info	11	prep work	29	artifacts	2	inter	2		1	info xfer	3	1	####	####	#NULL!
2	3	3	122	dynamic conditions	2	pt care	10	trust	42	standard	3	inter	2		1	info pull	2	2	1	0	1
2	3	3	123	coord	1	pt info	11	prep work	29	artifacts	2	inter	2		1	info xfer	3	1	1	1	2
2	3	3	124	human error	3	lapse	4	pt status	38		1	inter	2		1	info xfer	3	1	0	1	1
2	3	3	125	coord	1	pt info	11	prep work	29	artifacts	2	intra	4		1	info pull	2	3	1	0	1
2	3	3	126	coord	1	pt care	10	awareness	4	standard	3	inter	2		1	info xfer	3	2	1	0	1
2	3	3	127	coord	1	pt care	10	med order	17		1	inter	2		1	info pull	2	1	1	1	2
2	3	3	128	coord	1	contactability	2	noone to answer phone	22		1	inter	2		1		1	1	####	####	#NULL!
2	3	3	129	coord	1	pt status	12	schedule	40		1	inter	2		1	info xfer and pull	4	4	2	2	4
2	3	3	130	coord	1	pt status	12	awareness	4	standard	3		1		1	info pull	2	2	0	1	1
2	3	3	131	coord	1	pt status	12	pt transfer	39	standard	3	inter	2		1	info pull	2	2	1	1	2
2	3	3	132	coord	1	pt info	11		1	standard	3	inter and intra	3		1	info pull	2	4	0	1	1
2	3	3	133	coord	1	pt care	10	z_tests	49	standard	3	intra	4		1		1	1	1	0	1
2	3	3	134	coord	1	pt care	10	pt transfer	39		1	inter	2		1		1	2	1	1	2
2	3	3	135	coord	1	pt info	11	form	12	artifacts	2	inter and intra	3		1	info xfer	3	3	0	1	1
2	3	3	136	dynamic conditions	2	pt info	11	prep work	29	artifacts	2	intra	4		1	info pull	2	1	0	1	1
2	3	3	137	coord	1	pt info	11	blue card	6	artifacts	2	inter and intra	3		1	info pull	2	5	1	1	2
2	3	3	138	coord	1	contactability	2	noone to answer phone	22		1	inter	2		1		1	1	####	####	#NULL!
2	3	3	139	dynamic conditions	2	pt care	10	schedule	40	standard	3	inter and intra	3		1		1	4	####	####	#NULL!
2	3	3	140	coord	1	pt care	10	schedule	40	artifacts	2	inter	2		1	info pull	2	3	2	1	3

Hospital	phase	location_num	ID	type	type_num	Theme	theme_num	trigger	trigger_num	tangibility	tangibility_num	scale	scale_num	salience	salience_num	repair	repair_num	cost	d1	d2	d_total
2	3	3	141	coord	1	pt info	11	form	12	artifacts	2	inter	2		1	info xfer	3	4	####	####	#NULL!
2	3	3	142	coord	1	pt care	10	pt transfer	39		1	inter	2		1		1	2	1	1	2
2	3	3	143	coord	1	pt care	10	z_staffing	48		1		1		1		1	####	####	####	#NULL!
2	3	3	144	coord	1	pt care	10	patient	27	standard	3	inter	2		1	info xfer and pull	4	2	1	1	2
2	3	3	145	coord	1	pt care	10	med order	17	standard	3		1		1	info xfer and pull	4	4	####	####	#NULL!
2	3	3	146	coord	1	pt care	10	trust	42		1	inter	2		1	info xfer	3	1	1	0	1
2	3	3	147	coord	1	pt status	12	pt transfer	39	standard	3	inter	2		1	info pull	2	3	1	1	2
2	3	3	148	dynamic conditions	2	pt care	10	patient	27		1		1		1	info xfer	3	1	1	0	1
2	3	3	149	coord	1	pt info	11	prep work	29	artifacts	2	inter	2		1	info xfer	3	1	1	1	2
2	3	3	150	coord	1	pt info	11	prep work	29	artifacts	2	inter	2		1	info xfer	3	6	3	1	4
2	3	3	151	dynamic conditions	2	pt care	10	schedule	40	standard	3	inter	2		1	info pull	2	3	1	1	2
2	3	3	152	coord	1	pt care	10	pt transfer	39	standard	3	inter	2		1	info pull	2	3	1	1	1
2	3	4	1	coord	1	pt info	11	prep work	29	artifacts	2	inter and intra	3		1		1	####	1	0	1
2	3	4	2	coord	1	pt care	10	prep work	29	artifacts	2	inter and intra	3	explicit	2	info xfer	3	1	3	0	3
2	3	4	.	human error	3	pt care	10	pt coord	33	standard	3	inter and intra	3		1	info pull	2	5	1	0	1
2	3	4	3	coord	1	pt care	10	schedule	40	standard	3	inter and intra	3	explicit	2	info pull	2	13	4	1	5
2	3	4	.	coord	1	pt care	10	pt transfer	39	standard	3	inter	2	implicit	3	info pull	2	5	####	1	#NULL!
2	3	4	4	dynamic conditions	2	pt care	10	patient	27		1	inter and intra	3		1	info xfer	3	4	2	1	3
2	3	4	5	human error	3	pt care	10	pt coord	33	standard	3	inter and intra	3		1	info pull	2	4	2	0	2
2	3	4	6	coord	1	pt info	11	prep work	29	artifacts	2	inter	2		1	info pull	2	5	3	2	5
2	3	4	7	coord	1	pt care	10	schedule	40		1	inter	2		1	info xfer	3	7	1	1	2
2	3	4	8	coord	1	pt status	12	pt transfer	39	standard	3	inter	2		1		1	2	1	0	1
2	3	4	9	coord	1	pt care	10	schedule	40		1	inter and intra	3		1	info xfer	3	3	1	3	4
2	3	4	10	dynamic conditions	2	pt care	10	schedule	40		1	inter	2		1	info xfer	3	####	2	####	#NULL!
2	3	4	11	coord	1	pt status	12	awareness	4	standard	3	inter and intra	3		1	info pull	2	3	1	0	1
2	3	4	12	dynamic conditions	2	pt care	10	schedule	40		1	inter	2		1	info xfer	3	6	1	3	4
2	3	4	13	coord	1	pt info	11	prep work	29	standard	3	inter and intra	3		1	info pull	2	1	1	0	1
2	3	4	14	human error	3	lapse	4	pt status	38	artifacts	2	inter	2		1	info pull	2	2	1	1	2
2	3	4	15	coord	1	pt care	10	pt coord	33	standard	3		1		1	info xfer	3	1	1	0	1
2	3	4	16	coord	1	pt info	11	prep work	29	standard	3	inter and intra	3		1	info xfer and pull	4	6	2	1	3
2	3	4	17	coord	1	pt care	10	schedule	40	standard	3	intra	4		1	info pull	2	2	1	0	1
2	3	4	18	human error	3	slip	4	pt status	38	standard	3	inter	2		1	info pull	2	1	1	1	2
2	3	4	19	coord	1	pt care	10	pt status	38	artifacts	2	inter and intra	3		1		1	3	0	0	0
2	3	4	20	coord	1	pt info	11	prep work	29	artifacts	2	inter and intra	3		1		1	####	1	0	1
2	3	4	21	dynamic conditions	2	equipment	15	device	10		1	intra	4		1	info xfer	3	2	0	2	2
2	3	4	22	dynamic conditions	2	pt care	10	med order	17	standard	3	intra	4		1	info pull	2	2	1	1	2
2	3	4	23	dynamic conditions	2	pt care	10	schedule	40		1	inter and intra	3		1	info xfer	3	7	2	2	4
2	3	4	24	coord	1	pt info	11	prep work	29	artifacts	2	inter and intra	3		1		1	####	1	1	2
2	3	4	25	coord	1	pt info	11	prep work	29	artifacts	2	inter and intra	3		1		1	6	1	0	1
2	3	4	26	coord	1	pt care	10	blood	5	standard	3	inter	2		1	info pull	2	1	1	1	2
2	3	4	27	coord	1	pt care	10	schedule	40		1	inter and intra	3		1	info xfer	3	3	1	3	4
2	3	4	28	coord	1	pt care	10	trust	42	standard	3	inter	2		1	info pull	2	6	1	1	2
2	3	4	29	dynamic conditions	2	pt care	10	schedule	40		1	inter and intra	3		1	info xfer	3	2	1	2	3
2	3	4	30	coord	1	pt care	10		1		1	intra	4		1	info xfer	3	1	1	0	1
2	3	4	31	coord	1	pt info	11	prep work	29	artifacts	2	inter and intra	3		1		1	####	1	1	2
2	3	4	32	coord	1	pt care	10	schedule	40	artifacts	2	inter and intra	3		1	info pull	2	2	2	1	3
2	3	4	33	coord	1	pt care	10	prep work	29	artifacts	2	inter and intra	3		1	info xfer and pull	4	2	1	1	2
2	3	4	34	coord	1	pt care	10	med order	17	standard	3	inter and intra	3		1	info xfer	3	1	2	1	3
2	3	4	35	dynamic conditions	2	pt care	10	schedule	40		1	inter and intra	3		1		1	3	1	3	4
2	3	4	36	dynamic conditions	2	pt care	10	schedule	40		1	inter and intra	3		1		1	3	1	3	4
2	3	4	37	dynamic conditions	2	pt care	10	patient	27		1	inter and intra	3		1	info pull	2	5	1	2	3
2	3	4	38	dynamic conditions	2	pt care	10	schedule	40		1	inter and intra	3		1		1	3	1	3	4
2	3	4	39	dynamic conditions	2	pt care	10	patient	27		1	inter and intra	3		1	info xfer	3	3	2	1	3
2	3	4	40	coord	1	pt care	10	prep work	29	standard	3	intra	4		1	info pull	2	2	1	2	3
2	3	4	41	dynamic conditions	2	pt care	10	schedule	40		1	inter	2		1	info xfer and pull	4	6	3	2	5
2	3	4	42	coord	1	pt care	10	prep work	29	standard	3	intra	4		1		1	1	1	0	1
2	3	4	43	coord	1	pt care	10	pt status	38		1	inter	2		1	info pull	2	1	1	0	1
2	3	4	44	dynamic conditions	2	pt care	10	patient	27		1	inter and intra	3		1	info pull	2	3	1	2	3
2	3	4	45	coord	1	pt info	11	prep work	29	artifacts	2	intra	4		1	info xfer	3	2	1	0	1
2	3	4	46	coord	1	pt care	10	schedule	40		1	inter and intra	3		1	info pull	2	17	1	2	3
2	3	4	47	dynamic conditions	2	pt care	10	schedule	40		1	inter and intra	3		1		1	3	1	3	4
2	3	4	.	coord	1	pt info	11	form	12	artifacts	2	inter and intra	3		1	info pull	2	9	2	2	3
2	3	4	.	human error	3	slip	4	mysis	21	artifacts	2	inter and intra	3		1	info pull	2	9	2	2	3

Hospital	phase	location_ num	ID	type	type_num	Theme	theme_ num	trigger	trigger_num	tangibility	tangibility _num	scale	scale_num	salience	salience_num	repair	repair_ num	cost	d1	d2	d_total
2	3	4	49	coord	1	pt info	11	prep work	29	artifacts	2		1		1		1	1	2	1	3
2	3	4	50	dynamic conditions	2	pt care	10	schedule	40		1	inter	2		1	info xfer	3	1	0	2	2
2	3	4	51	coord	1	pt info	11	prep work	29	standard	3	intra	4		1		1	####	1	0	1
2	3	4	52	coord	1	pt care	10	pt transfer	39	standard	3	inter	2		1	info xfer	3	2	1	1	2
2	3	4	53	coord	1	pt care	10	pt transfer	39		1	inter	2		1	info xfer	3	3	1	1	2
2	3	4	54	coord	1	pt care	10	pt status	38	standard	3	inter	2		1	info pull	2	1	1	0	1
2	3	4	.	coord	1	pt care	10	med order	17	standard	3	inter and intra	3		1	info xfer	3	1	2	1	3
2	3	4	.	coord	1	pt care	10	prep work	29	standard	3	intra	4		1		1	1	1	0	1
2	3	4	56	coord	1	pt care	10	trust	42	standard	3		1		1	info pull	2	6	2	1	3
2	3	4	57	dynamic conditions	2	pt care	10	patient	27	standard	3		1		1	info pull	2	1	####	2	#NULL!
2	3	4	58	coord	1	pt care	10	prep work	29	artifacts	2		1		1	info pull	2	3	0	1	1
2	3	4	59	coord	1	pt info	11	prep work	29	artifacts	2	inter and intra	3		1	info xfer	3	4	0	2	2
2	3	4	60	dynamic conditions	2	pt care	10	schedule	40		1	inter and intra	3		1	info xfer and pull	4	12	1	3	4
2	3	4	61	coord	1	pt care	10	prep work	29		1	inter	2		1	info xfer and pull	4	1	2	1	3
2	3	4	62	dynamic conditions	2	pt care	10	schedule	40		1	inter	2		1	info pull	2	2	2	1	3
2	3	4	.	dynamic conditions	2	pt care	10	schedule	40		1	intra	4		1	info pull	2	3	1	1	2
2	3	4	.	coord	1	pt care	10	pt transfer	39	standard	3	inter	2		1	info pull	2	2	####	####	#NULL!
2	3	4	64	coord	1	pt status	12	awareness	4	standard	3	inter	2		1	info pull	2	1	1	0	1

B.3 Recorded breakdowns

Table 30 . Number of breakdowns recorded in Hospital_1 and Hospital_2.

	Hospital_1, Phase 1	**Hospital_1, Phase 2**	**Hospital_2**
Breakdowns total	68.00	166.00	162.00
Avg breakdowns per hour	1.45	3.20	2.89
Avg at Admissions	1.51	3.32	3.34
Avg at OR desk	1.27	3.67	2.44
Avg at Holding	0.83	1.62	2.86

B.4 Comparison of breakdowns according to their occurrence in each hospital

Table 31. Breakdowns distribution for each parameter in the coding scheme. Hospital_1 breakdowns are cumulative of Phase 1 and Phase 2.

Breakdown	value	hosp1	hosp2	n1	n2	CI	z-score	P (2-tailed)	Significance	Notes
type	coord	61.1%	60.5%	234	162	0.95	0.120	0.904		
	dynamic cond	23.1%	33.3%	234	162	0.95	2.241	0.025	Significant	more breakdowns due to dynamic conditions
	human error	9.4%	4.9%	234	162	0.95	1.666	0.096		same
	technical	6.4%	1.2%	234	162	0.95	2.516	0.012	Significant	less technical problems in a bigger and busier unit
theme	human factor	11.1%	3.1%	199	162	0.95	2.868	0.004	Significant	This difference may be due to observational limitatons - not all HF issues are observable behavior
	contactability	4.5%	4.3%	199	162	0.95	0.092	0.927		same
	pt care	57.3%	64.8%	199	162	0.95	1.451	0.147		same
	pt info	14.1%	16.7%	199	162	0.95	0.683	0.495		same
	pt status	7.5%	9.3%	199	162	0.95	0.616	0.538		same
	technical	5.5%	1.9%	199	162	0.95	1.761	0.078		same
tangibility	artifacts	43.3%	37.6%	150	93	0.95	0.878	0.380		same
	standards	56.7%	62.4%	150	93	0.95	0.878	0.380		same
trigger	awareness	10.9%	8.1%	128	123	0.95	0.755	0.450		same
	patient	11.7%	8.9%	128	123	0.95	0.729	0.466		same
	prep work	31.3%	24.4%	128	123	0.95	1.218	0.223		same
	pt transfer	11.7%	10.6%	128	123	0.95	0.277	0.782		same
	schedule	32.0%	43.9%	128	123	0.95	1.943	0.052		same, though a bit higher at h2, due to dynamic conditions
	trust	2.3%	4.1%	128	123	0.95	0.812	0.417		no sign difference in level of trust (phase 2 trust bkdwns excluded)
scale	inter	61.4%	45.4%	223	141	0.95	2.990	0.003	Significant	
	inter and intra	35.4%	44.0%	223	141	0.95	1.641	0.101		same
	intra	3.1%	10.6%	223	141	0.95	2.934	0.003	Significant	more breakdowns affected intra-team work
repair	info pull	46.7%	48.0%	199	127	0.95	0.229	0.819		same
	info push	50.3%	37.4%	199	127	0.95	2.282	0.022	Significant	less push at h2 due to dynamic conditions and lack of formal communication structure
	both	3.0%	12.6%	199	127	0.95	3.371	0.001	Significant	higher at h2

B.5 Comparison of breakdowns in Phase 1 & Phase 2

Table 32. Breakdowns distribution in Phase 1 & Phase 2.

Breakdown	value	phase1	phase2	n1	n2	CI	z-score	P-value		notes
type	coord	63.20%	60.20%	68.00	166.00	0.95	0.427	0.335		
	dynamic cond	22.10%	23.50%	68.00	166.00	0.95	0.231	0.409		
	human error	4.40%	11.40%	68.00	166.00	0.95	1.669	0.048		
	technical	10.30%	4.80%	68.00	166.00	0.95	1.561	0.059		
theme	human factor	8.10%	10.40%	62.00	163.00	0.95	0.519	0.302		validity - remained the same
	pt care	56.50%	48.50%	62.00	163.00	0.95	1.072	0.142		
	pt info	17.70%	10.40%	62.00	163.00	0.95	1.484	0.069		validity - remained the same
	pt status	11.30%	26.40%	62.00	163.00	0.95	2.434	0.007	Significant	increased bec. of coding as breakdowns what before was the usual case and was supposed to disappea
	technical	6.50%	4.30%	62.00	163.00	0.95	0.683	0.247		validity - remained the same
tangibility	artifacts	48.80%	41.10%	43.00	107.00	0.95	0.861	0.195		
	standards	51.20%	58.90%	43.00	107.00	0.95	0.861	0.195		
trigger	awareness	27.00%	2.90%	37.00	136.00	0.95	4.776	0.000	Significant	reduced due to intro of whiteboard
	prep work	29.70%	21.30%	37.00	136.00	0.95	1.075	0.141		validity - remained the same
	pt transfer	5.40%	9.60%	37.00	136.00	0.95	0.804	0.211		remained same despite wb
	schedule	37.80%	19.90%	37.00	136.00	0.95	2.269	0.012	Significant	may be due to seasonal diff- winer vs fall affects bed shortage in hospital
	trust	0.00%	27.90%	37.00	136.00	0.95	3.636	0.000	Significant	new breakdowns
	use-errors	0.00%	7.40%	37.00	136.00	0.95	1.705	0.044		new breakdowns
scale	inter	60.30%	61.90%	63.00	160.00	0.95	0.221	0.413		
	inter and intra	36.50%	35.00%	63.00	160.00	0.95	0.211	0.416		
	intra	3.20%	3.10%	63.00	160.00	0.95	0.039	0.485		
repair	info pull	44.80%	49.60%	58.00	135.00	0.95	0.612	0.270		
	info push	55.20%	50.40%	58.00	135.00	0.95	0.612	0.270		

B.6 Top 10% highest cost breakdowns

Table 33. Data subset of the top 10% highest cost breakdowns. The field 'safety' indicates if the breakdown had the potential to threaten patient safety (0=no threat, 1=threat to safety)

Hospital	phase	ID	type	theme	trigger	tangibility	scale	repair	cost	safety
1	1	31	coord	pt care	materials	standard	intra	info pull	32	0
1	1	33	conditions	pt care	schedule		intra	info xfer	20	0
1	2	122	dynamic cc	pt care	schedule		inter and intra	info xfer	17	0
1	1	24	coord	pt care	schedule		intra	info xfer	14	0
1	2	74	dynamic cc	pt care	schedule		inter	info xfer	13	0
1	2	90	dynamic cc	pt care	schedule		inter and intra	info pull	13	0
1	2	30	dynamic cc	pt care	patient		inter and intra	info xfer	12	0
1	2	133	dynamic cc	pt care	patient		inter and intra	info xfer	12	0
1	2	51	coord	pt care	schedule		inter	info xfer	11	1
1	2	98	dynamic cc	pt care	schedule		inter and intra	info xfer and pul	11	0
1	2	107	dynamic cc	pt care	schedule		inter and intra	info xfer	11	0
1	2	74a	dynamic cc	pt care	schedule		inter	info xfer	11	0
1	1	2	coord	pt info	prep work	artifacts	inter	info xfer	10	0
1	1	4	conditions	pt care	schedule		intra	info xfer	10	0
1	1	59	coord	pt info	prep work	artifacts	inter	info xfer	10	0
1	2	68	dynamic cc	pt care	schedule		inter and intra	info xfer	10	0
1	2	141	dynamic cc	pt care	schedule		inter and intra	info xfer and pul	10	0
1	2	61a	coord	pt info	prep work	artifacts	inter	info xfer	10	0
1	1	28	conditions	ity	late for		inter	info xfer	9	0
1	1	32	conditions	pt care	schedule		intra	info xfer	9	0
1	2	1	coord	pt info	prep work	standard	inter	info xfer	9	0
1	2	32	coord	pt info	prep work	artifacts	inter	info xfer	9	0
2	3	102	dynamic cc	pt care	schedule		inter and intra	info xfer	34	1
2	3	102b	coord	pt care	prep work	standard	inter and intra	info xfer	24	1
2	3	93	dynamic cc	pt care	schedule	standard	inter and intra		18	0
2	3	46	coord	pt care	schedule		inter and intra	info pull	17	0
2	3	109	coord	pt status	awareness	standard	inter and intra	info pull	14	0
2	3	3	coord	pt care	schedule	standard	inter and intra	info pull	13	0
2	3	60	dynamic cc	pt care	schedule		inter and intra	info xfer and pul	12	0
2	3	81	dynamic cc	pt care	schedule		inter and intra	info pull	10	0
2	3	87	dynamic cc	pt care	schedule			info xfer and pul	10	0
2	3	91	dynamic cc	pt care	schedule		inter	info xfer and pul	10	0
2	3	83	coord	pt care	schedule		intra		9	1
2	3	48a	coord	pt info	form	artifacts	inter and intra	info pull	9	1
2	3	48b	human err	slip	mysis	artifacts	inter and intra	info pull	9	0
2	3	97	coord	pt care	schedule				8	1

B.7 Highest cost breakdowns and safety

Table 34. Comparison of top 10% highest cost breakdowns between Hospital_1 and Hospital_2 in terms of potential for safety threat. 0=no threat and 1 = threat to safety.

safety	hosp1	hosp2	n1	n2	CI	z-score	P (2-tailed)	
1	4.55%	35.71%	22	14	0.95	2.446	0.014	Significant
0	95.45%	64.29%	22	14	0.95	2.446	0.014	Significant

Appendix C

C.1 Information flow diagrams

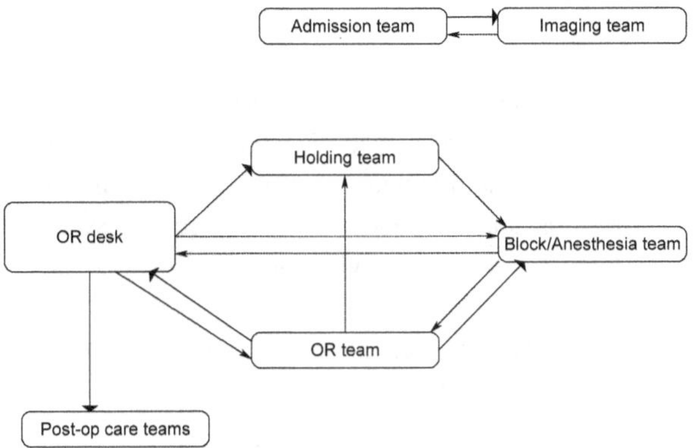

Figure 37: Day of surgery information flow model for Hospital_1, Phase_2. Solid arrows represent allowable phone communication between teams on any type of information exchange (*e.g.* patient status, schedule, OR readiness etc.). Dashed arrows represent allowable phone communication between teams on the theme of *patient status* only. The direction of the arrow indicates the receiving end of the phone communication.

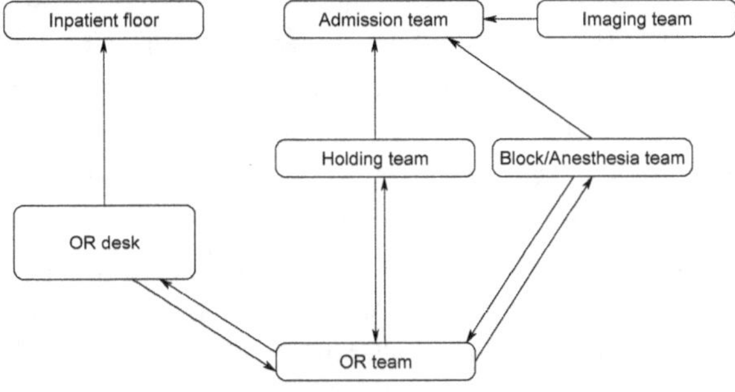

Figure 38: Day of surgery information flow model for Hospital_2. Dashed arrows represent allowable phone communication between teams on a particular theme only (*e.g.* patient status, schedule, staffing coordination, OR status, INpt status, OUTpt status). The theme for each arrow in the figure is defined in Table 26. The direction of the arrow indicates the receiving end of the phone communication.

Appendix D

D.1 Breakdown management in non-healthcare industries

For the purpose of defining a direction for future work in addressing large-scale coordination breakdowns in surgical patient care, a review of the successful approaches adopted in other industries is necessary. The literature discussing the management of breakdowns is dispersed. To identify a broad range of approaches, the following briefly summarizes work from the domains of aviation, reliability engineering, production and manufacturing, software and systems engineering. The focus of the methodologies review is on the systemic level, beyond cognitively-based human error analyses. Further, the aim is to review prospective, or predictive, approaches to breakdown management rather than accident-triggered retrospective methodologies.

Safety-critical domains

Two major strands of research span the approaches to breakdown management in safety-critical domains – work from the aviation industry and work from the reliability engineering domain.

Aviation

Breakdowns in group dynamics and in communication have been recognized as a major reason for aviation disasters [295]. In fact, one study found that over 70% of accidents occurred due to coordination and communication problems [167]. Massive research has been devoted to the management of breakdowns in aviation. The major outcome of this work is the development and evolution of the Crew Resource Management (CRM) programs, which build on the human error management framework and on previous work concerning the design of procedures that ensure safety operations. Research on accident cause factors established that deviation from basic operational procedures was the principal contributing factor behind a large number of aircraft accidents [167]. On the other hand, procedure application as rule-following has been shown to affect actual in-situ practice by encouraging procedure modifications due to the inability of procedures to cope with all types of unexpected situations [76, 111]. Thus, the core concept in aviation behind both procedure design and CRM is strict adherence to established standards of operation, while allowing flexibility of action in their execution. Most importantly, procedure design and CRM standards are to be based on an inside-out understanding of the context in-use, *i.e.* on the end-user's needs.

Design of procedures

Procedures in aviation are defined as specifications prescribing progression of sub-tasks and actions to ensure that the primary task will be carried out efficiently, logically, and without error. A procedure should also promote coordination between agents in the system - cockpit crew, cabin crew, ground crew, and others [75]. Procedures specify unambiguously what the task is, when it is conducted and in what sequence, by whom, how it is executed and what type of feedback is provided. Thus, procedures support teamwork, communication, and division of labor.

Procedures are standardized in order to establish common ground among individual crew members who are not familiar with each other's experience and technical skills – a standard creates a common mental model of everyone's roles and thus coordinates the cooperative activity. The belief is that through Standard Operating Procedures (SOPs) the replacement of a crew member in-flight with another qualified member will be a seamless and safe process.

A procedure establishes boundaries of allowable behavior. Flexibility in executing procedures is important and thus personal practices that express individualism and creativity without violating procedural constraints are considered conforming behaviors. Further, formal open feedback channels are established so that front-line crew can provide input on procedure adequacy and propose modifications. The NASA guidelines on the design of fligh-deck procedures fall in five broad categories: flexibility within boundaries, continuous procedure improvement "inside-out", systems approach, context-specific design, and clarity [75]. The list of relevant guidelines in each of these categories from the NASA document can be found in Appendix D.2.

In aviation, compliance with procedures is considered paramount. At the same time, appreciation for the dynamic nature of the work and environment has resulted in integrating flexibility through allowing individualism and creativeness in the execution of procedures within boundaries. Procedures provide a *baseline* [75], they are a resource for action [76]. The role of flight management is to provide the best possible baseline for the flight crews.

The majority of guidelines resound the necessity for procedure design with a systems approach and focus on contextual factors in the end user's environment. The notion of continuous improvement of operating procedures is also significant. Formal channels of communication are established in order to allow front-line workers to effect improvement of practice.

Crew resource management

Extending the scope of safety-oriented procedure design, CRM training programs adopted in aviation, as well as in other industries, focus on optimizing communication and coordination by capitalizing on knowledge of human error factors. Error management, or CRM, is based on understanding the nature and extent of error, changing the conditions that induce error, determining behaviors that prevent or mitigate error, and training personnel in their use [132]. Specific CRM techniques are discovered beyond the training programs – they are developed by trial and error, as well as by observations of others [75]. Similar to procedures, the CRM techniques serve as a resource for action and adherence is expected. Some techniques are standardized as SOPs.

The core stance of CRM training is that errors in work environments are imminent. There are three lines of defense to manage errors: avoid them, trap them before they are committed, and mitigate their consequences [130]. The three countermeasures to errors, including breakdowns, clearly reflect the idea that no errors should be allowed to propagate through the system.

Avoid errors. Although all errors cannot be avoided, their incidence can be reduced through utilization of communication tools that ensure standardized communication with the goal to maintain situational awareness among all agents. The key tools to achieve error avoidance are: briefings, checklists, call-outs, double-checks, procedures, and phraseology.

Trap errors. Techniques of communication facilitate the correction of an error that has occurred. Such techniques are checking and then verifying information, confirming communications (*i.e.* closing the information flow loop), clarifying communications to resolve ambiguities, questioning and communication of suspicious conditions.

Mitigate error consequences. A culture with high value on teamwork and leadership creates an environment that mitigates the consequences of errors by promoting all individuals to contribute to problem identification and resolution, and by reducing the effects of power dynamics. All crew members carry responsibility to voice concerns and contribute to solutions. Procedures are established to promote communication between pilots and co-pilots and to facilitate leadership assignment in situations of conflicting views on flight plan.

The CRM error management approach is premised on the idea that organizations will communicate their formal understanding of errors and the fact that errors will occur, and they will adopt a non-punitive approach to errors [129, 132]. Errors and breakdowns are treated as resources for improvement and culture – national, professional and organizational – promotes norms of compliance with SOPs [129]. *Trust* regarding a shared commitment to safety between management and crew members is required. Even though a causal relationship between safety and CRM has not been established, the implementation of CRM programs in aviation has been shown to promote desirable behavioral changes [249] and has been associated with safety improvements [131].

CRM and procedures

One of the objectives of any procedure is to promote better coordination among crews. System procedures, accordingly, are shared and conducted by all agents. To benefit from the knowledge of CRM, procedure design takes into account human factors issues in order to promote crew coordination. For example, reducing variance allows crews to effectively and efficiently execute important operational tasks with minimal need for formal co-coordination and superfluous communication [115, 150]. Reducing variance in functional tasks allows other agents a better chance at monitoring the task during critical phases of work. Flexible techniques can be positively introduced during non-critical phases. In defining a procedure, the crew coordination requirements for the respective context must be defined [75].

Reliability engineering

The term reliability is founded on the concept of failure. Reliability engineering is commonly understood as the application of methodologies that ensure the engineering of a system void of failures. Reliability engineering is a scientific approach to the analysis of expected or actual reliability of a complex system, and the identification of actions to reduce failures or mitigate their effect. Typically, engineers utilize predictive reliability tools, monitor and analyze field failures, and suggest design changes. The overall goal of reliability engineering is to make processes more reliable in order to reduce repairs and lower costs. The reliability engineering practice spans various domains, including aviation, train operations, automotive industry, software engineering, etc.

One of the most important initial design stages in reliability engineering is failure analysis This analysis aims at the understanding and prediction of all potential failure conditions of the system and their consequences. The focus during failure analysis is on prevention of failure during design – not on the correction of failure during operations. Techniques, some predictive and others retrospective in nature, are employed in order to assess the probability and severity of potential failures and to develop barriers early in the design cycle.

Predictive failure analysis

Failure Mode and Effects Analysis (FMEA) is one of the first steps in a system reliability approach [141]. FMEA examines potential failures of a system in a formalized fashion, identifying their causes, assessing their effects on the system and probabilities of occurrence. Process FMEA involves reviewing an exhaustive number of the process components to identify any process failures that may occur.

Questions addressed are: how can each component fail, what mechanisms can produce the failures, what will the effects of the failure be, does the failure threaten safety, how is the failure detected, what provisions does the design provide to compensate for the failure. The severity of each failure is then categorized as one of: catastrophic, critical, marginal, and negligible. Design of countermeasures is considered. The probability of occurrence is similarly determined as frequent, probable, occasional, remote, and extremely unlikely. A criticality index is computed which, along with the severity classification, determines the priority for failure prevention. Following FMEA, design activities are centered around failure cause removal, thus decreasing the probability of occurrence and reducing the severity of failure. One of the major goals of an FMEA analysis, besides reliability, is the early identification of system problems that prevents costly changes at later stages of the design process [278]. FMEA is a popular tool for reliability analysis and is a recommended practice by several engineering standards: MIL-STD-1629, IEC 812, SAE ARP 926, IEEE std. 352.

Fault Tree Analysis (FTA) is another predictive method of failure analysis that uses deduction to quantify the probability of occurrence of an accident through fault tree and failure data [141]. The system reliability is determined through known probabilities of each potential failure. Since FTA is a top-down approach where failure modes are the starting point of analysis, the output produced from an FMEA analysis can serve as input to the FTA efforts [278]. Given a failure mode, all system factors that could potentially contribute to the failure are identified. All combinations of latent and proximal factors are considered, reflecting a holistic systemic approach. Both qualitative and quantitative analysis of the fault tree are performed. Simulations are utilized in the probabilistic analysis and the importance factor for each contributing event is estimated. The main contributing factors to failure are identified based on occurrence rates and estimation, and design for failure prevention is implemented.

A variety of derivative techniques from the FMEA and FTA exist and are commonly applied in the analysis of reliability of systems – with each approach expanding the scope of analysis in a direction of interest. For example, the Advanced Cause Consequence Analysis (ACCA) looks at potential breakdowns and failures similarly to the FMEA, quantifies the probability of their occurrence as the FTA, and examines the existing and potential types of barriers in the system that affect the probability of breakdowns [135]. Another instance of the predictive analysis approach is the Hazard and Operability Studies (HAZOP). This approach implements a set of guide-words to more formally systematize the analysis of potential breakdowns and their consequences.

Design of barriers

With the goal to control breakdowns and failures and maximize reliability, system designers provide the socio-technical system with a set of barriers. A barrier is a technical or human support that protects the socio-technical system from the occurrence or consequences of undesirable events [283]. It is an obstacle that may either prevent an action from being carried out or an event from taking place, or prevent or lessen the impact of the consequences [139]. In this sense, the notion of a barrier reflects the prevention and avoidance approach utilized in aviation. Barriers protect the system with respect to criteria such as safety, workload, quality [283].

Similarly to the three-tier approach of CRM in aviation, the design of barriers falls into three equivalent levels of failure management: prevention, correction and containment [283]. Prevention barriers support the anticipation of failure. Correction barriers support the recovery from, interruption and stopping of failure. Containment barriers aim to mitigate consequences.

Barriers can be classified according to their function into four broad categories [139]:

- *Material barriers* – such as walls, doors, or equipment use – physically prevent an event from occurring or limit its negative consequences (some approaches refer to such barriers as *physical barriers* [135]).
- *Functional barriers* – such as a door key or a password – establish logical and temporal links between an action and an operation by setting a pre-condition to the operation.
- *Symbolic barriers* – such as warning signs – indicate a limitation on actions and require interpretation. As they do not establish a pre-condition, these barriers can be disregarded by the agents of the system.
- *Immaterial barriers* – such as norms, procedures and organizational restrictions – are the formal and informal rules for action that are not physically present during an operation but are expected to be known by the system agents. (Immaterial barriers are also referred to as *procedural barriers* [135]).

An additional class of barriers, used in accident analyses is *circumstantial barriers*. These are the unintended/unplanned favorable circumstances that prevent a breakdown from occurring [135].

Barrier identification to particular system design is usually carried out in an informal fashion – by looking at known barriers implemented in other systems' processes [139]. Re-analysis through the predictive techniques (*i.e.* FMEA), or simulations, evaluate the effectiveness of the implemented barriers. The barrier validation may identify the need for modification or additional barrier design.

Barrier failures are also considered. Some of the essential requirements for barrier effectiveness are a valid design specification, verified implementation, reliable functioning and high compliance by users.

Safety: flexibility and standardization

Rules, or standards of practice, are essential to coordinate processes and integrate the functions of an organization. Rules reduce the amount of variance, uncertainty, and complexity in everyday work. However, rules restrict individual autonomy and are sometimes inadequate, which leads to their modification in the work practice. A central problem in the management of safety and coordination in organizations is to establish the proper balance between flexibility and standardization [111]. In safety-critical domains, the presence of both is crucial in order to avoid over-reliance on standards or the lack of explicit coordination in unexpected situations. A lack of degree of liberty can also encourage agents to modify procedures in order to make them more flexible and applicable.

Rules fall into three categories [116]: goal rules that prescribe the goals to be achieved without specifying actions, procedural process rules that define high-level procedures to reach decisions about a course of action, and action rules that prescribe a specific course of actions to be taken. These categories showcase the property of rules to vary in the degree of flexibility they allow. It has been suggested that different types of rules are needed for different processes within an organization, thus optimizing flexibility and autonomy, while maintaining safety within the critical processes [111].

One way to work towards establishing the balance between flexibility and standards is for rules to clearly specify system boundaries of safe operation and suggest ways of handling system states close to those boundaries [235]. Rules are defined in terms of the specific constraints of the work practice. In this way, the flexibility introduced to the system would not undermine safety. This concept is reflected in the guidelines for procedure design in aviation where a procedure is mostly regarded as a resource for action – allowing flexibility and individualism in its execution and setting a *window of opportunity* for the timing of the enactment [75]. As such, procedures fall within the procedural rules category – they provide guidance and opportunity for flexible action. Procedural rules have indeed been recommended for the safety-critical domains [116]. Goal rules are also advocated as facilitators of flexibility within boundaries [235].

A complementary approach to striking a balance between flexibility, standards and safety is to promote the role of good adaptive skills of front-line agents. Adaptation is considered a critical cognitive skill in the face of unexpected situations – one has to balance the risks, current conditions, potential outcomes, larger goals and constraints that operate on the situation [76]. Investing in developing people's skill at adaptation at system boundaries is considered beneficial to safety. It is recommended that the type of work and environment be considered when determining the level of the organization where rules should be defined [116]. For predictable systems, action rules are best made at high levels of the organization. In innovative work environments, rules are best made at operative levels. When there are interactions among multiple organizational units, the rules and standards should be established at high levels.

Other domains

The problems of breakdown management have also been addressed in industries that are not concerned with safety, such as operations management, software engineering, and systems engineering.

Operations management

Zero-defects processes

In the context of organizational operations, one company is known as the epitome of both efficiency and reliability – Toyota. The Toyota Production System (TPS) is based on several principles to produce an integrated socio-technical system. At the core of the TPS approach lies the idea of eliminating inconsistency and waste from the production process by rigidly scripting production flows. This tightly scripted production process is coupled with a high level of flexibility that allows continuous improvement in the processes. The main wastes addressed by the TPS are transportation of products or motion of agents, overproduction, waiting of operator or machine, over-processing, inventory, defects and re-work. The goal is to produce perfect first-time quality and to minimize waste. When an error occurs, the production line is stopped, the error is analyzed and a solution is sought so that no error propagation would result in a final imperfect product. Strategies such as load leveling, production flow and visual control contribute to the accomplishment of smooth efficient operations. However, the success of Toyota has been attributed not to the tools and methodologies, which have been replicated elsewhere without the same success, but to the unique cultural perspective of continuous learning and improvement, which is implicitly regulating the work at Toyota [263, 264].

Behind a rigidly specified activity in terms of content, sequence, timing and outcome is the notion that the execution of the activity is a test for the validity of the prescribed procedure. If the outcome is not as expected, one has to determine whether the procedure is inadequate to produce the outcome or the person performing the procedure is not able to perform it correctly. Because each task has a prescribed measurement for success, the task can be tested like a hypothesis, giving rise to the use of the scientific method. In this sense, the view of highly specified procedures is one of scientific experimentation where a procedure is the outcome of a rigorous problem-solving process that requires a detailed assessment of the current state of affairs and a well-substantiated plan for improvement and expected outcome. And like a hypothesis, these improved procedures will be subjected to the test of practice [263]. To distance the approach from casual speculation about outcomes, the anticipated results of the solution are quantified and performance is tested against the expectation [264].

To minimize waste and optimize efficiency, every employee-employee connection and every product or information flow at Toyota follows a simple and direct path (while each path is not dedicated to a single product) that is standardized and unambiguous. When an employee makes a request, there is a specific way to state the need and a specific person designated to take responsibility of further processing of the need. Thus, variance and miscommunication are prevented and requests are handled smoothly [263]. This is in contrast to other companies where needs for assistance are expected to be met based on who is available at the moment of the request, which often results in no person taking responsibility. At Toyota, the number of workers per team is determined by the types of problems expected to occur and the level of assistance the team members need. The determination of team size and labor allocation is also subject to the scientific method – if assistance is not delivered within an allotted time criterion, then the procedure specification hypothesis is false and the system needs to be improved. Also, if work in practice reveals that workers contact people other than those in the designated direct links, then it will be concluded that the actual demand or capacity does not match expectations. Thus, the system will be evaluated and improved.

Employees at Toyota are not explicitly trained to apply the scientific approach to their work. They discover the implicit rules through problem solving, led by their supervisors. Supervisors promote the scientific thinking by encouraging employees to critically evaluate the work they are performing and the processes that are used. With this approach, Toyota encourages and expects improvement ideas to originate from front-line workers, with the assistance and coaching of managers [263]. Toyota managers act as coaches, enablers and teachers because lower-level workers are better able to observe and experiment with the actual production. This approach contrasts with many other companies where only managers solve problems. Further, higher levels of management can propose adequate problem solutions only following direct observation of the work practice

[264] and having included front-line workers in the change process [263].

In summary, the TPS thrives on strict compliance with unambiguously specified procedures of work as much as it also promotes continuous procedure improvement that stems from the lowest organizational level. A scientific approach to problem definition, change and outcome planning, and change testing in practice underlies the continuous improvement culture that aims to accomplish the goals of minimum waste, optimal efficiency and zero failures.

Process design

A common approach to process (re-)design is to identify redundant and non-value added steps, or areas where tasks spend long idle periods before they are worked on, and to modify the process to address these problems [118, 120]. A very popular method, applied in a variety of domains, reflecting this approach is a derivation of the Toyota Production System - Lean Management. Similar to the TPS, the fundamental concept is to identify waste and inefficiencies in a process and to create solutions that improve operations to a value-optimal workflow. Each process step is analyzed with respect to the criteria for value towards the final product, and non-value steps are eliminated. The optimization of product flow and elimination of waste is through standardization of processes and the involvement of all employees in process improvement. The implementation of Lean programs is preceded by a culture change as the existing paradigms of meaningful work necessarily change through the Lean framework. Lean culture emphasizes interdisciplinary teams, managers as enablers, rewards group sharing and information sharing, and is process driven. These values are in contrast to traditional organizational culture where managers direct, rewards are to individuals, information is guarded and experts drive the organization.

Coordination theory adopts a different focus in that it recommends replacing coordination mechanisms with alternative ones. Coordination problems arise from dependencies that constrain the performance of tasks. Once the specific problematic dependencies and associated coordination mechanisms are identified, alternative coordination mechanisms can be considered [68]. Dependencies relate to the tasks performed and the resources associated with tasks. Therefore there are three types of dependencies that can be established in a process: task-task, task-resource, and resource-resource. To identify process dependencies and coordination mechanisms, one can examine the current coordination mechanisms and determine the dependencies they manage. Another method is to list the activities and resources in the process, identify the dependencies and then determine how they are managed. A third approach is to look for problematic areas in the process and then identify the underlying dependencies.

Variance analysis is another well-established method for socio-technical process (re-)design. Variance is defined as an unexpected or unwanted deviation from standard operating conditions or specifications [222]. Hence, the construct of variance is reflective of the breakdown concept. Variance analysis starts with the identification of key variances, *i.e.* those that can have serious consequences. A table of key variance control is generated that shows the manner, the location, and the functional role associated with possible detection, correction, and prevention of each key variance [72, 220]. Having identified those mechanisms that need to be changed, variance analysis recommends redesigning the work system in a way that increases control and autonomy at the sources of variance. The (re-)design is determined based on analysis of the skills, knowledge, information and authority need to the effective control of variances.

Regardless of the approach, when dramatic levels of improvement are required, re-engineering the entire work process is recommended as it allows to break away from current conventions of practice and the constraints of organizational boundaries [117]. In process re-design, issues of re-focusing the work must be addressed so that task management overhead is prevented by removing liaisons, interfaces and some mechanisms of coordination. Ideally, those who use the output of a process will be the ones performing the process. In addition, parallel activities must be linked, rather than their results integrated – thus, creating stronger dependency between the activities. Finally, process re-engineering principles advise the continuous learning paradigm where front-line workers should be empowered with decision-making in regards to their work. In addition, formal channels of communication with management are established to facilitate the improvement efforts.

Software engineering

The later in the software development lifecycle an error is discovered, the more expensive it is to fix it [71, 180, 216]. This is due to the fact that at later stages, not only the error necessitates repair, but also the designs and implementations that followed as a result of the latent error. Detecting and repairing an error at the requirements stage costs five to ten times less than fixing it at the coding stage, and 20 times less than fixing it at the maintenance stage [172]. The cost of repair would usually entail redesign, re-coding, rewriting documentation and replacing software in the field [70, 172]. On average 40% of total project budget could be spent on rework [236]. As a result, the focus in error management within software engineering is on prevention and early detection [196], rather than mitigation of consequences. Prevention and early detection of software-related errors are enabled by efforts targeted at the requirements stage [70], one of the very early development stages in the software lifecycle. Development process related errors are addressed by promoting communication between development teams [180].

Requirements management is a systematic approach to eliciting, organizing, documenting and managing the initial and the changing requirements of a system [172]. The primary output of these efforts is the development of requirements specifications that define the complete external behavior of the system to be built. Rigorous requirements management is recommended as one method of reducing error costs – the core idea being that identifying and fixing errors as early in the process as possible reduces cost associated with repair and with multiplier effects. The goal of requirements specifications is to be accurate, complete and unambiguous. To accomplish this, the process of requirements management must follow extensive analysis of the end-user environment and population. The first step is the elicitation of requirements through a systematic approach of data collection – expert and end-user interviews, facilitator-managed workshops, and in-situ observations. Next, the requirements are defined through an iterative process of re-definition until the requirements set is clear, complete, consistent and provides traceable information. Predictive failure/breakdown analysis is conducted at this point to produce a further set of requirements, specifically addressing potential problematic situations. The requirements are then organized in various categories that facilitate the division of labor among engineering teams – e.g. hardware and software categories. Design, implementation and testing decisions are made and added to resulting documents. The resulting hierarchy of requirements and implementation documents – the requirements specification – includes a complete description of functional and non-functional requirements.

The software development process itself has been shown to facilitate the occurrence of errors, specifically in safety-critical aspects. Safety-related software errors in complex distributed systems have been found to result from *lack of communication between development teams* and misunderstandings related to the interactions of various software-software and software-hardware interfaces [180, 216] (*i.e.* interoperability issues). To prevent such breakdowns and errors, it has been recommended that [180]:

For communication among engineering teams

- Informal communication among teams should be promoted
- Changes in requirements should be communicated clearly and in a timely fashion to all teams that may be affected

For safety-critical software concerns

- Focus should be on the interfaces between the software and the system in analyzing the problem domain
- Safety-critical hazards should be identified early in the requirements analysis
- Include requirements for defensive design (i.e. barriers)

It has also been suggested that communication issues among development teams resulting in safety-critical software errors can be addressed by means of performing a large-scale FMEA that spans all safety-critical software components, *i.e.* on each side of software/hardware interfaces [216]. Thus, the FMEA analysis will examine the information themes that are usually the subject of inter-team breakdown.

Systems engineering

Systems engineering is a holistic and interdisciplinary approach to the design and management of systems that is concerned with large and complex socio-technical systems. When dealing with large systems, the issues of logistics and coordination of different micro-systems can become difficult and systems engineering addresses those by the employment of technical, process and human-centered approaches. The scope of systems engineering is the processes of design, development, production and operation of complex systems. Systems engineering is driven by the recognition that in large-scale engineered systems accident mechanisms go beyond proximate events and pure engineering activities [174]. Hence, system safety engineering should account for the social system – structure, management, procedures, and culture, in addition to the technology being designed.

As was the case with software engineering, efforts at discovering and validating the system requirements are essential. Methods that allow early detection of possible failures are integrated into the design process as well. In fact, safety concerns are addressed even before system architecture and requirements are elicited [174]. However, what really distinguishes the design of large complex systems is the multidisciplinary approach to a large design problem, which results in methods that more thoroughly investigate system requirements from multiple perspectives, thus providing a more holistic view of the problems of design.

In regards to factors contributing to accidents, systems engineering looks at dysfunctional interactions among the micro-systems of a socio-technical system and at lack of appropriate safety constraints [174]. Constrains must enforce safety as related to the physical, social, and organizational aspects of the system domain. One of the primary factors of consideration is the coordination among multiple agents and micro-systems, especially when there is an overlap area or boundary area where two or more agents control the same process [173]. It has been suggested that such dysfunction can be related to the amount of distance between the levels separating workers in the departments from a common manager – the greater the distance, the more difficult the communication, thus the greater the risk [174]. Hence, the goals for addressing safety from a systems engineering perspective should account for such latent factors that are not usually covered by other error/accident analysis models and the goals of analysis should be to [174]:

- Expand accident analysis by forcing consideration of factors other than component failures and human errors
- Include system design errors and dysfunctional micro-system interactions in analysis
- Shift the focus from the role of human error in accidents to the mechanisms and factors that shape human behavior (*i.e.* the context)
- Shift the focus from causes of accidents to reasons for accidents
- Examine the processes involved in accidents, not just the events and conditions

To address these goals from the initial stages of design, standards have been established. The comprehensive exploration of requirements-related issues is covered by the stakeholder concern-oriented approach to architectural system descriptions (*e.g.* std. IEEE 1471 and ISO/IEC 42010, and [151]). It has been suggested that the application of architecting concepts facilitates the attainment of increased quality, usability, flexibility, reliability, interoperability, etc. A system architecture is the structure of components, their interrelationships, and the principles and guidelines governing their design and evolution. Architecting contributes to the development, operation, and maintenance of a system from its initial concept until its retirement from use. System architecture potentially impacts all processes within the system life cycle. The stakeholder concerns approach to system architecting addresses the early conceptualization of system (re-)design.

Every system is considered in the context of its environment – developmental, technological, business, operational, organizational, political, regulatory, social and any other influences upon the setting and circumstances surrounding the system development and integration are accounted for [183]. The environment is modeled through the lens of the stakeholders of the system and the architectural concerns they hold for that system. Identifying the stakeholders helps the architect to get a detailed understanding of the context in which the system must be developed, used and operated. Stakeholders include the client for the system, its users, operators, maintainers, system developers, suppliers, regulators, etc. The focus on stakeholders reflects the reality that a multitude of functional roles are involved in complex systems, with each person having a different concern with respect to the system.

Concerns represent the interests and values of stakeholders with respect to their involvement with the system. Concerns may be requirements-oriented or design-oriented [182] – *e.g.* safety, performance, reliability, security, information sharing, etc. Concerns are the root of the process of decomposition into requirements

[197]. Once the stakeholders are identified, their concerns are examined, incorporated in the architecture, and systematically addressed through the system design. The rationale for key decisions made is also documented. The resulting architectural description is considered complete when it has covered the system through all the stakeholder concerns [182].

Human-centered approaches to systems design, such as ISO/TR 18529 and others, reflect equivalent ideas to those described above (*i.e.* IEEE 1471 and ISO/IEC 42010). The latter were chosen for discussion since they are more comprehensive in the recommended analysis by adding the concern dimension and providing specific guidelines for materializing the concerns (which are beyond the scope of this review). What is important to note is that both the human-centered and the concern-oriented methods focus on addressing the interests of all stakeholders early in the design of a system, thereby minimizing potential inter-team issues in system development and in system integration.

Summary of breakdown management approaches

A common trend in breakdown management amongst the industries reviewed is the focus on active prevention rather than reactive treatment. The breakdowns and error management philosophy for all of the domains reviewed is underpinned by the idea to remove the causes of problems as early as they can possibly be anticipated. Given that aviation workers deal with higher levels of uncertainty in their daily operations compared to engineers from the other domains, the recognition that breakdowns will occur has resulted in formalized methodologies for their reactive management as well. Especially important for the mitigation and avoidance of breakdowns in aviation is the idea of minimization of power dynamics through formalized communication procedures. While most industries emphasize the significance of strict compliance with established procedures, they also appreciate the need for flexibility and autonomy in people's work. Thus, process designers aim to embed flexibility in various ways within procedural work – *e.g.* through time boundaries, system boundaries, or a continuous improvement philosophy with the aim to achieve a problem-free optimal process. Although the tools used to address breakdowns differ among the industries, a common tendency is to provide a non-punitive environment with formal channels of communication between workers and management in order to facilitate improvements initiated by front-line staff. As far as design of procedures or systems is concerned, a common strategy is the investment in comprehensive analysis during initial planning and requirements gathering, so as not to allow breakdowns and errors to propagate to later stages of design.

All of the industries reviewed adopt a systemic approach to the management of breakdowns. However, the most elaborate and specific is the systems engineering method of eliciting requirements from all system stakeholders by identifying and addressing each stakeholder's concerns. Systems and software engineering also provide for special attention to interactions among micro-systems, at system interfaces – whether they are human-computer, software-software, or software-hardware interfaces.

Table 35 summarizes the important features of the breakdown management approaches of the industries reviewed in this chapter.

Table 35. Breakdown management in selected industries.

Industry / Value	Aviation	Reliability Engineering	Operations Management	Software Engineering	Systems Engineering
main focus	• prevention • avoidance • mitigation	prevention	prevention (zero failures)	prevention	prevention
flexibility through	time boundaries	system boundaries	continuous improvement	N/A	N/A
compliance through	SOPs	barriers	• highly specified procedures • standardized work	N/A	safety constraints
tools	• SOPs • formal channels of communication • non punitive culture • mitigation of errors through culture change • CRM	• barriers • flexible rules • FMEA, FTA, ACCA, etc.	• scientific approach to in-situ problem solving and testing • formal channels of communication • eliminate non-value activities • replace problematic coordination mechanisms • LEAN, Six Sigma, Variance analysis	• inter-team communication • rigorous requirements through in-situ work • barriers • IEEE830	• comprehensive descriptions of stakeholder concerns • dysfunctional component interactions • continuous attention to evolving concerns • stakeholder requirements • early evaluation • IEEE1471, STAMP, etc.
context specific design	compatibility of procedure and end-user environment	N/A	driven by front-line workers	N/A	consider all stakeholders and system context influences
systems approach	• all agents involved in design • document design logic • no error propagation	• all agents and system components considered • no error propagation • balance between flexibility and standards	• any change effects through the system are considered • no error propagation	• no error propagation • focus on interfaces	• all stakeholders • all system components interactions • environmental influences

Table 35 (Cont'd).

Industry / Value	Aviation	Reliability Engineering	Operations Management	Software Engineering	Systems Engineering
error management philosophy	• avoid, trap, mitigate • reduce effect of power dynamics	remove causes of errors	• shorten distance between process output and execution • control breakdowns at their source • re-engineer work to avoid errors	prevent error by investing in initial requirements efforts	avoid breakdowns through common language about the system with all stakeholders
scope	• management • end user feedback • crew coordination requirements	early requirements and specifications	• end-user driving continuous improvement • process driven (not expert)	• early requirements and specifications • inter-team communication	• early system design • dysfunctional component interactions • focus on context

D.2 NASA guidelines on the design of fligh-deck procedures [75]

Flexibility within boundaries

- For every task on the flight deck, there is a time boundary. This period is sometimes referred to as the *window of opportunity*, indicating the time period in which a task can take place. A well managed crew schedules the required tasks within a window of opportunity in a way that it will not be done too early or too late.
- Over-proceduralization will have an adverse effect on the practices and outcomes. Having too many procedures creates a false sense of security, leads to an inflexible system, and results in procedure violations.

Continuous procedure improvement "inside-out"

- Management, though the feedback loop should be watchful of techniques that are used on the line. Techniques that conform to procedures should not be interfered with. Techniques that have a potential for procedure deviation should be addressed. Techniques that yield better and safer ways of doing a task may be considered for SOP.

Systems approach

- When introducing new technology into the cockpit, the procedure designer should reevaluate all of the existing procedures and policies in light of the new technology and support the new technology via new procedures.
- System procedures involve cockpit and aircraft crew, ground crew, management and air traffic control. Such system procedures must be developed using a systems approach – developing a common definition of the task and involving all the components of the system in the design of the procedure. If the piecemeal approach is taken, the foundations of a potential breakdown are laid.
- Not only the principal participants of a system, but also others that are affected should be involved and informed in the design and modifications of a system procedure.
- The entire documentation supplied to the cockpit (and elsewhere) should be regarded as a system, and designed accordingly as a system, not a collection of independent documents. A clear and logical (from the user's view) structure for this system and a criterion for the location of different procedures is important. An effective index in each manual would go a long way toward aiding pilots in finding materials they seek, especially when it is an unfamiliar, obscure, or seldom accessed procedure.
- The SOP documentation should not only explain the mechanics of the procedure, but also state the logic behind it. A detailed account of the operational logic, and system constraints should be part of the documentation.

Context-specific design

- Procedures must be tailored to the particularities of the type of operation. Ignoring these particularities can foster low compliance with procedures on the line.
- Paperwork should be designed carefully to be compatible with the device for which it is intended. Particular care should be exercised in preparing materials for computer based

systems. It may be necessary to provide differently formatted documents for different cockpit configurations.

- Particular attention should be paid in order to safeguard information transfer during critical and high workload phases of flight. Callouts should be economical, unambiguous, and should convey only the information needed by the other crew member(s). They should not distract the crew member from his primary task(s).
- Procedure designers should always bear in mind the contribution which any procedure makes to total workload of the crew at any given time. They should be especially sensitive to procedures that may require crew attention in times of high workload, and should strive to "manage" workload by moving tasks that are not time-critical to periods of low workload.

Clarity

- If the same procedure can yield significantly different outcomes, then the procedure must be modified in order to eliminate its embedded ambiguity. A procedure should lead to a totally predictable outcome.

References

1. *Fluorouracil incident root cause analysis*, Institute for Safe Medication Practices. May 2007: Toronto, Canada.

2. *Human Factors Engineering and Preferred Practices for the Design of Medical Devices . ANSI/AAMI HE48*. 1993, Association for the Advancement of Medical Instrumentation (AAMI).

3. *Improving Patient Care by Reporting Problems with Medical Devices: A MedWatch Continuing Education Article*. 1997, Food and Drug Administration (FDA). Available: http://www.fda.gov/downloads/Safety/MedWatch/UCM168502.pdf.

4. *Human centred design processes for interactive systems. ISO 13407*. 1999, International Organization for Standardization (ISO).

5. *Application of risk management to medical devices. ISO 14971*. 2000, International Organization for Standardization (ISO).

6. *Human-centred Lifecycle Process Descriptions. ISO/IEC TR 18529*. 2000, International Organization for Standardization (ISO).

7. *Human Factors Implications of the New GMP Rule. Overall Requirements of the New Quality System Regulation*. 2000, Food and Drug Administration (FDA). Available: http://www.fda.gov/MedicalDevices/DeviceRegulationandGuidance/PostmarketRequirements/HumanFactors/ucm119215.htm.

8. *Medical Device Use-Safety:Incorporating Human Factors Engineering into Risk Management*. 2000, Center for Devices and Radiological Health. The Food and Drug Administration (FDA).

9. *Human Factors Design Process for Medical Devices. ANSI/AAMI HE74*. 2001/(R)2009, Association for the Advancement of Medical Instrumentation (AAMI).

10. *AHRQ's Patient Safety Initiative: Building Foundations, Reducing Risk. Interim Report to the Senate Committee on Appropriations.*, 04-RG005,

A.P.N., Editor. 2003, Agency for Healthcare Research and Quality (AHRQ). Available: http://www.ahrq.gov/qual/pscongrpt/.

11. *Closed Claim Report. Data Sharing Project.* 2003, Physician Insurers Association of America (PIAA)

12. *Building a Better Delivery System: A New Engineering/Health Care Partnership*, ed. Reid, P.P., Compton, W.D., Grossman, J.H. & Fanjiang, G. National Academies Press, Washington, DC (2005)

13. *Going Lean in Health Care*, in *IHI Innovation Series white paper*. 2005, Institute for Healthcare Improvement: Cambridge, MA. Available: Available on www.IHI.org.

14. *The American Heritage® Medical Dictionary*. Houghton Mifflin Company (2007)

15. *Improving America's Hospitals: The Joint Commission's Annual Report on Quality and Safety*. 2007, Agency for Healthcare Research and Quality (AHRQ). Available: http://www.jointcommission.org/Library/annual_report.

16. *Medical devices -- Application of usability engineering to medical devices. ISO/IEC 62366.* 2007, International Organization for Standardization (ISO).

17. *World Aliance for Patient Safety. WHO guidelines for safe surgery.* 2008, World Health Organization.

18. *Human factors engineering – Design of medical devices. ANSI/AAMI HE75.* 2009, Association for the Advancement of Medical Instrumentation (AAMI).

19. *Electronic Health Record Usability: Vendor Practices and Perspectives.* 2010, Agency for Healthcare Research and Quality (AHRQ). Available: http://healthit.ahrq.gov/portal/server.pt/gateway/PTARGS_0_3882_913591_0_0_18/EHRVendorPractices&Perspectives.pdf.

20. *Many Errors by Medical Residents Caused by Teamwork Breakdowns, Lack of Supervision*, in *Press Release*. October 22, 2007, Agency for Healthcare Research and Quality (AHRQ): Rockville, MD.

21. Adachi, W., Lodolce, A.E., Use of failure mode and effects analysis in improving the safety of i.v. drug administration. *Am J Health Syst Pharm*, 2005. 62(9): p. 917-920.

22. Adamson, J., *Combined qualitative and quantitative designs*, in Ebrahim, A.B.S. (ed.): *Handbook of health research methods. Investigation, measurement and analysis*. Open University Press, Berkshire, UK (2005) p. 230-245.

23. Andrews, L.B., Stocking, C., Krizek, T., Gottlieb, L., Krizek, C., Vargish, T.,

Siegler, M., An alternative strategy for studying adverse events in medical care. *The Lancet*, 1997. 349(9048): p. 309-313.

24. Ash, J. S., Berg, M., Coiera, E., Some unintended consequences of information technology in health care: the nature of patient care information system-related errors. *Journal of the American Medical Informatics Association*, 2004. 11(2): p. 104-112.

25. Ash, J.S., Sittig, D.F., Campbell, E., Guappone, K., Dykstra, R.H. An unintended consequence of CPOE implementation: shifts in power, control, and autonomy. in *Proc AMIA*. 2006.

26. Ash, JS, Sittig, DF, Poon, EG, Guappone, K, Campbell, E, Dykstra, RH, The Extent and Importance of Unintended Consequences Related to Computerized Provider Order Entry. *JAMIA*, 2007. 14: p. 415-423.

27. Baker, G.R., Norton, P.G., Flintoft, V., Blais, R., Brown, A., Cox, J., et al., The Canadian Adverse Events Study. *Can. Med. Assoc. J*, 2004. 170 (11): p. 1678-86.

28. Bannon, L.J., Bødker, S., *Beyond the interface: encountering artifacts in use*, in Caroll, J. (ed.): *Designing interaction: psychology at the human-computer interface*. Cambridge University Press (1991) p. 227-253.

29. Bardram, J.E., Temporal Coordination: On Time and Coordination of CollaborativeActivities at a Surgical Department. *Computer Supported Cooperative Work*, 2000. 9: p. 157-187.

30. Barley, S. R., The Alignment of Technology and Structure through Roles and Networks. *Administrative Science Quarterly*, 1990. 35(1): p. 61-103.

31. Barley, Stephen R., Technology as an Occasion for Structuring: Evidence from Observations of CT Scanners and the Social Order of Radiology Departments. *Administrative Science Quarterly*, 1986. 31(1): p. 78-108.

32. Barnard, P., May, J., Duke, D., Duce, D., Systems, Interactions and Macrotheory. *ACM Trans. Comput.-Hum. Interact.*, 2000. 7: p. 222-262.

33. Basnyat, S, Palanque, P. A Task Pattern Approach to Incorporate User Deviation in Task Models. in *1st ADVISES Young Researchers Workshop*. 2005. Liege, Belgium.

34. Basu, A., Blanning, R.W., A Formal Approach to Workflow Analysis. *Information Systems Research*, 2000. 11(1): p. 17-36.

35. Bates, D. W., Spell, N., Cullen, D.J., Burdick, E., Laird, N., Petersen, L., Small, S.D., Sweitzer, B.J., Leape, L.L., The Costs of Adverse Drug Events in Hospitalized Patients. *JAMA*, 1997. 277(4): p. 307-311.

36. Belford, T., *Captain Picard to surgery, please: Voice-operated badges - just like on Star Trek - give busy nurses an edge in patient care*, in *The Globe and Mail*. Nov. 27, 2007: Toronto.

37. Bellorini, A., Vanderhaegen, F. . Communication and cooperation analysis in air traffic control. in *Int Symp Aviation Psych* 1995. Columbus, OH.

38. Benn, J.; Healey, A.N.; Hollnagel, E., Improving performance reliability in surgical systems. *Cogn Tech Work*, 2008. 10(4): p. 323--333.

39. Berkowitz D.A., Barnett G.O., Chueh H.C. eWhiteBoard: a real time clinical scheduler. in *AMIA*. 1999. Washington, DC.

40. Bogner, M.S. (ed.), *Human error in medicine.* Lawrence Erlbaum, Hillsdale NJ (1994)

41. Bogner, M.S. (ed.), *Misadventure in health care.* Lawrence Erlbaum, Hillsdale NJ (2003)

42. Boyatzis, R., *Transforming qualitative information: Thematic analysis and code development.* Sage Publications, Thousand Oaks, CA (1998)

43. Braun, Virginia and Clarke, Victoria, Using thematic analysis in psychology. *Qualitative Research in Psychology*, 2006. 3(2): p. 77 - 101.

44. Brennan, T. A., Leape, L. L., Laird, N. M., Hebert, L., Localio, A. R., Lawthers, A. G., Newhouse, J. P., Weiler, P. C., Hiatt, H. H., Incidence of adverse events and negligence in hospitalized patients: results of the Harvard Medical Practice Study I. *Qual Saf Health Care*, 2004. 13(2): p. 145-151.

45. Calland, J.F., Guerlain, S., Adams, R.B., Tribble, C.G., Foley, E., Chekan, E.G., A systems approach to surgical safety. *Surg Endosc*, 2002. 16(6): p. 1005-1014.

46. Callantine, T. , *Activity tracking for pilot error detection from flight data*, 2002-211406, N.C.R., Editor. 2002.

47. Cannon-Bowers, J., Salas, E., Converse, S., *Shared mental models in expert team decision making*, in N. J. Castellan, J. (ed.): *Individual and group decision making*. Erlbaum, Hillsdale, NJ (1993) p. 221-246.

48. Casey, S., *Set Phasers on Stun and other true tales of design, technology and human error.* 2 ed. Aegean Publishing, Santa Barbara CA (1998)

49. Catchpole, K, Giddings, A, Hirst, G, Dale, T, Peek, G, De Leval, M., A Method for Measuring Threats and Errors in Surgery. *Cogn Tech Work*, 2008. 10(4): p. 295-304.

50. Catino, M., Blame culture and defensive medicine *Cogn Tech Work*, 2009. 11(4): p. 245-253.

51. Chassin, M.R., Becher E.C., The Wrong Patient. *Ann Intern Med*, 2002. 136: p. 826-833.

52. Chassin, MR., Becher, EC., The Wrong Patient. *ANN INTERN MED*, 2002. 136(11): p. 826-833.

53. Christian, C. K., Gustafson, M.L., Roth, E. M., Sheridan, T. B., Gandhi, T. K., Dwyer, K., Zinner, M. J., Dierks, M. M., A prospective study of patient safety in the operating room. *Surgery*, 2006. 139(2): p. 159-173.

54. Clark, H.H., *Using Language*. Cambridge University Press, New York (1996)

55. Cockton, G., Woolrych, A., Sale Must End: should discount methods be cleared off HCI's shelves? *ACM Interactions* 2002. 9(5): p. 13-18.

56. Cohen, M.R. *An injustice has been done: Jail time given to pharmacist who made an error.* [cited July 22, 2010]; Available from: http://www.ismp.org/pressroom/injustice-jailtime-for-pharmacist.asp.

57. Coiera, E. Clinical Communication - A New Informatics Paradigm. in *Am Med Inf Assoc*. 1996.

58. Coiera, E., Tombs, V., Communication behaviours in a hospital setting: an observational study. *Brit Med J*, 1998. 316(7132): p. 673-676.

59. Coiera, Enrico, When Conversation Is Better Than Computation. *J Am Med Inform Assoc*, 2000. 7(3): p. 277-286.

60. Cole, M., Engestrom, Y., *A cultural historical approach to distributed cognition*, in Salomon, G. (ed.): *Distributed cognitons*. Cambridge University Press, Cambridge (1993) p. 1-46.

61. Colla, J. B., Bracken, A. C., Kinney, L. M., Weeks, W. B., Measuring patient safety climate: a review of surveys. *Qual Saf Health Care* 2005. 14(5): p. 364-366.

62. Collins, S.A., Currie, L., Patel, V.L., Bakken, S., Cimino, J.J. Multitasking by clinicians in the context of CPOE and CIS use. in *Proc MedInfo*. 2007. Brisbane, Australia.

63. Commission, The Joint. *Lessons Learned: Wrong Site Surgery*. 1998 [cited July 29, 2010]; Available from: http://www.jointcommission.org/SentinelEvents/SentinelEventAlert/sea_6.htm.

64. Cooper JB, Gaba DM, Liang B, Woods D, Blum LN., National Patient Safety Foundation agenda for research and development in patient safety. *MedGenMed*, 2000. 2(4).

65. Corcoran-Perry, S., Graves, J., Supplemental-information-seeking behavior of

cardiovascular nurses. *Research in Nursing & Health*, 1990. 13(2): p. 119-127.

66. Covell, D. G., Uman, G. C., Manning, P. R., Information Needs in Office Practice: Are They Being Met? *Ann Intern Med* 1985. 103(4): p. 596-599.

67. Creswell, J.W., *Research design: Qualitative, quantitative, and mixed methods approaches.* Sage Publications, Thousand Oaks, CA (2003)

68. Crowston, Kevin, A Coordination Theory Approach to Organizational Process Design. *Organization Science*, 1997. 8(2): p. 157-175.

69. Danieli, M. On the Use of Expectations for Detecting and Repairing Human-Machine Miscommunications. in *AAAI-96, Workshop on Detecting, Preventing and Repairing Human-Machine Miscommunications*. 1996. Portland, OR.

70. Davis, A., *Identifying and Measuring Quality in Software Requirements Specifications*, in *IEEE Int'l Metrics Symp*. 1993, IEEE CS Press, 141-152: Baltimore.

71. Davis, A., *Software Requirements, Objects, Functions, and States*. Prentice Hall, Englewood Cliffs, NJ (1993)

72. Davis, L. E., Wacker, G. J., *Job design*, in Salvendy, G. (ed.): *Handbook of human factors*. Wiley, New York, NY (1987) p. 431-452.

73. Day, S., Dalto, J., Fox, J., Turpin, M., Failure Mode and Effects Analysis as a Performance Improvement Tool in Trauma. *Journal of Trauma Nursing:*, 2006. 13(3): p. 111-117.

74. de Vries, E. N., Ramrattan, M. A., Smorenburg, S. M., Gouma, D. J., Boermeester, M. A., The incidence and nature of in-hospital adverse events: a systematic review. *Qual Saf Health Care*, 2008. 17(3): p. 216-223.

75. Degani, A., & Wiener, E. L., On the Design of Flight-Deck Procedures. *NASA Technical Memorandum #177642*, 1994. Moffett Field, CA: NASA Ames Research Center.

76. Dekker, S., Failure to adapt or adaptations that fail: contrasting models on procedures and safety. *Applied Ergonomics*, 2003. 34: p. 233-238.

77. DeRosier, J.M., Taylor, L. , *Analyzing missing patient events at the VA*, in *Topics in Patient Safety*. 2005, VA National Center for Patient Safety. Available: http://www.va.gov/ncps/TIPS/Docs/TIPS_NovDec05.pdf.

78. Dexheimer JW, Brown LE, Leegon J, Aronsky D., Comparing decision support methodologies for identifying asthma exacerbations. *Studies in Health Technology and Informatics*, 2007. 129(2): p. 880-884.

79. Dickson E.W., Singh S., Cheung D.S., Wyatt C.C., Nugent A.S. , Application of Lean Manufacturing Techniques in the Emergency Department. *J Emerg Med*, 2008. 37(2): p. 177-182.

80. Dourish, P. Implications for design. in *Proc CHI*. 2006. Montreal, Canada: ACM.

81. Drews, F.A. The frequency and impact of task interruptions on patient safety in the ICU. in *Proc Human Factors Erg Soc*. 2007.

82. Edmondson, A. C., Speaking Up in the Operating Room: How Team Leaders Promote Learning in Interdisciplinary Action Teams. *J Management Studies*, 2003. 40(6): p. 1419-1452.

83. Edmondson, A. C., Bohmer, R. M., Pisano, G. P., Disrupted Routines: Team Learning and New Technology Implementation in Hospitals. *Administrative Science Quarterly*, 2001. 46(4): p. 685-716.

84. Edwards, P.J., Jacko, J., Moloney, K.P., Sainfort, F. HCI Challenges Case Study: implementing an electronic medical record. in *CHI workshop*. 2006. Montreal, Canada.

85. Ellingsen, G., Monteiro, E. A patchwork planet - The Heterogeneity of electronic patient record systems in hospitals. in *IRIS*. 2000.

86. Emanuel L, Berwick D, Conway J, Combes J, Hatlie M, Leape L, Reason J, Schyve P, Vincent C, Walton M, *What exactly is patient safety?* , in Henriksen K, B.J., Keyes MA, Gandy ML (ed.): *Advances in Patient Safety: New Directions and Alternative Approaches*. Agency for Healthcare Research and Quality, Rockville, MD (2008) p. 19-36.

87. Engeström, R. Miettinen & R.-L-. Punamäki (Eds), *Perspectives on activity theory*. Cambridge University Press, Cambridge (1999)

88. Expert group on learning from adverse events in the NHS., *An Organisation With a Memory*. Department of Health. The Stationery Office, London (2000)

89. Fairbanks, R. J., Bisantz, A. M., Sunm, M., Emergency department communication links and patterns. *Ann Emerg Med*, 2007. 50(4): p. 396-406.

90. Faules, Don, The use of multi-methods in the organizational setting. *Western Journal of Communication*, 1982. 46(2): p. 150 - 161.

91. FDA, *Preproduction quality assurance planning: Recommendations for medical device manufacturers.*, Health, C.f.D.a.R., Editor. 1989, The Food and Drug Administration.

92. FDA, *Medical Device Use-Safety:Incorporating Human Factors Engineering into Risk Management*, Center for Devices and Radiological Health, Editor.

2000, The Food and Drug Administration.

93. Ferlie, E. B., Shortell, S. M., Improving the Quality of Health Care in the United Kingdom and the United States: A Framework for Change. *Milbank Quarterly*, 2001. 79(2): p. 281-315.

94. Fields, R., Paternò, F., Santoro, C., Tahmassebi, S., Comparing design options for allocating communication media in cooperative safety-critical contexts: a method and a case study. *ACM Trans. Comput.- Hum. Interact.*, 1999. 6: p. 370-398.

95. Fisne, J., What works: ER tracking systems prevent "lost" patients. *Health Mana Technol*, 1999. 20(10): p. 52-53.

96. Flach, P.A., *The geometry of ROC space: understanding machine learning metrics through ROC isometrics*, in *20th International Conference on Machine Learning (ICML'03)*. 2003, AAAI Press.

97. Flynn, E.A., Barker, K.N., Gibson, J.T., Pearson, R.E., Berger, B.A., Smith, L.A., Impact of interruptions and distractions on dispensing errors in an ambulatory care pharmacy. *Am. J. Health. Syst. Pharm*, 1999. 56(13): p. 1319--1325.

98. France D, Leming-Lee S, Jackson T, Feistritzer N, Higgins M, An observational analysis of surgical team compliance with perioperative safety practices after crew resource management training. *Am J Surg*, 2008. 195(4): p. 546-553.

99. Frohlich, D., Drew, P., Monk, A., Management of Repair in Human-Computer Interaction. *Human-Computer Interaction*, 1994. 9(3): p. 385 - 425.

100. Fu, L., Salvendy, G., Turley, L., Effectiveness of user testing and heuristic evaluation as a function of performance classification. *Behaviour & Information Technology*, 2002. 21(2): p. 137 - 143.

101. Gaba, David M., Anaesthesiology as a model for patient safety in health care. *Brit Med J*, 2000. 320(7237): p. 785-788.

102. Galliers, J., Wilson, S., Fone, J., A method for determining information flow breakdown in clinical systems . . *Int J Medical Informatics*, 2007. 76(S): p. 113-121.

103. Garbis, C. and Y. Waern, Team coordination and communication in a rescue command staff: The role of public representations. *La Travail Humain*, 1999. 62(3): p. 273-291.

104. Gefen, D., Karahanna, E., Straub, D.W., Trust and TAM in Online Shopping: An Integrated Model. *MIS Quarterly*, 2003. 27(1): p. 51-90.

105. Gittell, J.H., Organizing work to support relational co-ordination. *International Journal of Human Resource Management*, 2000. 11(3): p. 517-539.

106. Gittell, J.H., Fairfield, K.M., Bierbaum, B., Head, W., Jackson, R., Kelly, M., Laskin, R., Lipson, S., Siliski, J., Thornhill, T., Zuckerman J., Impact of relational coordination on quality of care, postoperative pain and functioning, and length of stay: a nine-hospital study of surgical patients. *Medical Care*, 2000. 38(8): p. 807-819.

107. Graban, Mark, *Lean Hospitals: Improving Quality, Patient Safety, and Employee Satisfaction*. CRC Press, New York (2009)

108. Greenberg, C.C., Regenbogen, S.E., Studdert, D.M., Lipsitz, S.R., Rogers, S.O., Zinner, M.J., Gawande, A.A., Patterns of Communication Breakdowns Resulting in Injury to Surgical Patients. *Journal of the American College of Surgeons*, 2007. 204(4): p. 533-540.

109. Grol, R. P., Bosch, M. C., Hulscher, M. E., Eccles, M. P., Wensing, M., Planning and Studying Improvement in Patient Care: The Use of Theoretical Perspectives. *Milbank Quarterly*, 2007. 85(1): p. 93-138.

110. Grote, G., Helmreich, R.L., Sträter, O., Häusler, R., Zala-Mezö, E., Sexton, B., *Setting the stage: characteristics of organizations, teams and tasks influencing team processes*, in R, D. (ed.): *Group interaction in high risk environments*. Ashgate (2004) p. 111-141.

111. Grote, G., Weichbrodt, J., Gunther, H., Zala-Mezo, E., Kunzle, B., Coordination in high-risk organizations: the need for flexible routines. *Cogn Tech Wrok*, 2009. 11: p. 17-27.

112. Grote, G., Zala-Mezö, E., Grommes, P., *The effects of different forms of coordination on coping with workload*, in R, D. (ed.): *Group interaction in high risk environments*. Ashgate (2004) p. 39-55.

113. Guerlain, S., Adams, R.B., Turrentine, F.B., Shin, T., Guo, H., Collins, S.R., Calland, J.F., Assessing team performance in the operating room: Development and use of a "black-box" recorder and other tools for the intraoperative environment. *Journal of the American College of Surgeons*, 2005. 200(1): p. 29-37.

114. Guerlain, S., Turrentine, F., Bauer, D., Calland, J., Adams, R., Crew resource management training for surgeons: feasibility and impact. *Cognition, Technology & Work*, 2008. 10(4): p. 255-264.

115. Hackman, J. R., *Teams, leaders, and organizations: New directions for crew-oriented flight training*, in E. L. Wiener, B.G.K., and R. L. Helmreich (ed.): *Cockpit resource management*. Academic Press, San Diego (1993) p.

116. Hale, A. R., Swuste, P., Safety rules: procedural freedom or action constraint? *Safety Science*, 1998. 29(3): p. 163-177.

117. Hammer, M., Re-engineering Work: Don't Automate, Obliterate. *Harvard Business Review*, 1990. 68(July/ August): p. 104-112.

118. Hammer, M., Champy, J., *Reengineering the corporation: a manifesto for business revolution*. Harper Business, New York (1993)

119. Hardstone, G., Hartswood, M., Procter, R., Slack, R., Voss, A., Rees, G., *Supporting informality: team working and integrated care records*, in *CSCW*. 2004, ACM: Chicago, Illinois, USA.

120. Harrington, H.J., *Business Process Improvement: the breakthrough strategy for total quality, productivity and competitiveness*. McGraw Hill, New York (1991)

121. Hartswood, M., Procter, R., *Design guidelines for dealing with breakdowns and repairs in collaborative work settings*. 2000, Academic Press. p. 91-120.

122. Hartswood, M., Procter, R., Rouncefield, M. Slack, R. Making a Case in Medical Work: Implications forthe Electronic Medical Record. in *CSCW*. 2003: Kluwer Academic Publishers.

123. Hassenzahl, M., Tractinsky, N., User Experience: A research agenda. *Behaviour and IT*, 2006. 25(2): p. 91-97.

124. Haynes, A. B., Weiser, T. G., Berry, W. R., Lipsitz, S. R., Breizat, AH. S., Dellinger, E. P., Herbosa, T., Joseph, S., Kibatala, P. L., Lapitan, M. C. M., Merry, A. F., Moorthy, K., Reznick, R. K., Taylor, B., and Gawande, A. A., A Surgical Safety Checklist to Reduce Morbidity and Mortality in a Global Population. *NEJM*, 2009. 360(5): p. 491-499.

125. Healey, A., Catchpole, K., Yule, S., Enhancing surgical systems. *Cognition, Technology & Work*, 2008. 10(4): p. 251-254.

126. Healey, A.N., Olsen, S., Davis, R., Vincent, C.A., A method for measuring work interference in surgical teams. *Cogn Tech Work*, 2008. 10(4): p. 305-312.

127. Healey, AN, Nagpal, K, Moorthy, K, Vincent, CA, Engineering the system of communication for safer surgery *Cogn Tech Work*, 2010. DOI: 10.1007/s10111-010-0152-5.

128. Helmreich, R. L., On error management: lessons from aviation. *BMJ*, 2000. 320(7237): p. 781-785.

129. Helmreich, R.L. . Error management as organisational strategy. in *IATA Human Factors Seminar* 1998.

130. Helmreich, R.L., & Merritt, A.C. , *Culture at work in aviation and medicine: National, organizational, and professional influences.* Ashgate., Aldershot, U.K (1998)

131. Helmreich, R.L. & Wilhelm, J.A., Outcomes of crew resource management training. *Int J Aviation Psychology*, 1991. 1: p. 287-300.

132. Helmreich, R.L., Merritt, A.C., & Wilhelm, J.A., The evolution of Crew Resource Management training in commercial aviation. *Int J of Aviation Psychology*, 1999. 9(1): p. 19-32.

133. Hendrich, A., Chow, M., Skierczynski, B.A., Lu, Z., A 36-Hospital Time and Motion Study: How. Do Medical-Surgical Nurses Spend Their Time? *The Permanente Journal*, 2008. 12(3).

134. Herfarth, C., Lean surgery through changes in surgical work flow *Brit J Surgery*, 2003. 90(5): p. 513-514.

135. Hessami, A.G. Foord, A.G, *Systems safety-a real example (European rail traffic management system, ERTMS)*, in *Int Conf Human Interfaces in Control Rooms, Cockpits and Command Centres.* 2001, (IEE Conf. Publ. No. 481) Manchester, UK.

136. Hoff, T., Jameson, L., Hannan, E., Flink, E., , A Review of the Literature Examining Linkages between Organizational Factors, Medical Errors, and Patient Safety. *Med Care Res Rev*, 2004. 61(1): p. 3-37.

137. Hollnagel, E., *The phenotype of erroneous actions: implications for HCI design*, in Weir, G., Alty, J. (ed.): *HCI and Complex Systems*. Academic Press, London (1991) p. 73-121.

138. Hollnagel, E., *Human reliability analysis: Context and control.* Academic Press, London (1993)

139. Hollnagel, E., *Accident and barriers*, in *EU Conf Cognitive Science Approaches to Process Control*. 1999: Villeneuve d'Ascq, France, 175–180.

140. Horsky, J., Zhang, J., Patel, V.L., To err is not entirely human: Complex technology and user cognition. *Journal of Biomedical Informatics*, 2005. 38(4): p. 264-266.

141. Hoyland, A., Rausand, M., *System reliability theory: models, statistical methods, and applications*. 2nd ed. John Wiley & Sons, Inc.(2004)

142. Hudson, P., Applying the lessons of high risk industries to health care. *Qual Saf Health Care*, 2003. 12(suppl 1): p. i7-i12.

143. IEEE Architecture Working Group I, *Recommended Practice for Architectural Description of Software-Intensive Systems: IEEE Std 1471-*

2000. IEEE(2000)

144. Institute of Medicine, *Crossing the Quality Chasm: A New Health System for the 21st Century*. National Academies Press, Washington, DC (2001)

145. Israelski, E.W., Muto, W.H., Human factors risk management as a way to improve medical device safety. *Joint Commission Journal on Quality and Safety*, 2004. 30: p. 689-95.

146. Israelski, E.W., North, R., Kaye, R., *Implementing Human Factors Principles and Best Practices in Medical Device Design: Lessons Learned*, in *Webinars on CD*. 2007, AAMI Publications.

147. Jacques, P., Minear, M., *Improving Perioperative Patient Safety Through the Use of Information Technology*: *Advances in Patient Safety: New Directions and Alternative Approaches*. Agency for Healthcare Research and Quality (2008) p.

148. JCAHO, *National Patient Safety Goal compliance trends—hospital. January 1, 2003–September 30, 2007*, Organizations, J.C.o.A.o.H., Editor.

149. Jens, H. Weber-Jahnke, Morgan, P. Engineering Medical Information Systems: Architecture, Data and Usability and Security. in *International Conference on Software Engineering - proc. companion*. 2007: IEEE Computer Society.

150. Johnston, A. N., *An introduction to airline operating procedures*, document, A.L.t., Editor. 1991, Dublin Ireland: Aer Lingus.

151. Kandé, M. M., *A concern-oriented approach to software architecture*. Doctoral dissertation. École Polytechnique Fédérale de Lausanne(2003)

152. Kaplan, B., Evaluating informatics applications - some alternative approaches. *Int J Medical Informatics*, 2001. 64: p. 39-56.

153. Kaptelinin, V., Nardi, B.A., *Activity theory: basic concepts and applications*, in *CHI '97 extended abstracts on Human factors in computing systems: looking to the future*. 1997, ACM: Atlanta, Georgia.

154. Karl, RC, Aviation. *Journal of Gastrointestinal Surgery*, 2009. 13(1): p. 6-8.

155. Karsh, B. T., Beyond usability: designing effective technology implementation systems to promote patient safety. *Qual Safety Health Care*, 2004. 13(5): p. 388-394.

156. Killich, S., Luczak, H., Schlick, C., Weissenbach, M., Wiedenmaier, S. and Ziegler, J., Task modelling for cooperative work. *Beh. & Info. Tech.*, 1999. 18: p. 325-338.

157. Kohn, L.T., Corrigan J.M., Donaldson M.S. (eds.), *To err is human: building*

a safer health system. National Academy Press, Washington DC (1999)

158. Kontogiannis, T., Malakis, S., A proactive approach to human error detection and identification in aviation and air traffic control. *Safety Science*, 2009. 47(5): p. 693-706.

159. Kopach-Konrad, R., Lawley, M., Criswell, M., Hasan, I., Chakraborty, S., Pekny, J., Doebbeling, B., Applying Systems Engineering Principles in Improving Health Care Delivery. *Journal of General Internal Medicine*, 2007. 22(0): p. 431-437.

160. Koppel, R., Metlay, J. P., Cohen, A.,Abaluck, B., Localio, A. R., Kimmel, S. E., Strom, B.L., Role of Computerized Physician Order Entry Systems in Facilitating Medication Errors. *JAMA*, 2005. 293(10): p. 1197-1203.

161. Kossiakoff, A., Sweet, W.N., *ystems Engineering Principles and Practice*. Wiley, New York, NY (2003)

162. Koutantji, M., McCulloch, P., Undre, S., Gautama, S., Cunniffe, S., Sevdalis, N., Davis, R., Thomas, P., Vincent, C., Darzi, A., Is team training in briefings for surgical teams feasible in simulation? *Cognition, Technology & Work*, 2008. 10(4): p. 275-285.

163. Kushniruk, AW, Triola, MM, Borycki, EM,Stein, B, Kannry, JL., Technology induced error and usability: The relationship between usability problems and prescription errors when using a handheld application. *International Journal of Medical Informatics*, 2005. 74(7-8): p. 519-526.

164. Kuutti, K, *Activity Theory as a potential framework for human- computer interaction research*, in Nardi, B. (ed.): *Context and Consciousness: Activity Theory and Human-Computer Interaction*. MIT Press (1996) p.

165. Lachiche, N., Flach, P.A., *Improving accuracy and cost of two-class and multi-class probabilistic classifiers using ROC curves*, in *20th International Conference on Machine Learning (ICML'03)*. 2003, AAAI Press.

166. Lasko, T.A., J.G. Bhagwat, K.H. Zou and Ohno-Machado, L., The use of receiver operating characteristic curves in biomedical informatics. *J Biomedical Informatics*, 2005. 38(5): p. 404–415.

167. Lautman, L., Gallimore, P.L., Control of the crew caused accident: Results of a 12-operator survey. *Boeing Airliner*, 1987. April–June: p. 1-6.

168. Law, E. L-C., Bevan, N., Christou, G., Springett, M. & Lárusdóttir, M. (Eds.): *Proc Int Workshop Meaningful Measures: Valid Useful User Experience Measurement (VUUM)* IRIT Press - Toulouse, France, Reykjavik, Iceland (2008) p.

169. Law, E. L-C., Hvannberg, E., & Hassenzahl, M. (Eds.). Proc Int workshop

Towards a Unified View of User Experience. in *in conj with NordiCHI*. 2006. Oslo, Norway: Available at: http://www.cost294.org/.

170. Leape, L., *Preventability of medical injury*, in Bogner, M.S. (ed.): *Human Error in Medicine*. Erlbaum, Hillside, NJ (1994) p.

171. Leape, L.L., Bates, D.W., Cullen, D.J., Cooper, J., Demonaco, H.J., Gallivan, T., et al., Systems Analysis of Adverse Drug Events. *JAMA*, 1995. 274(1): p. 35-43.

172. Leffingwell, D., Davis, A., Requirements Management in Medical Device Development. *Medical Device and Diagnostic Industry Magazine*, 1996. 18(3): p. 100-116.

173. Leplat, J., *Occupational Accident Research and Systems Approach*, in J. Rasmussen, K.D., and J. Leplat (ed.): *New Technology and Human Error*. John Wiley & Sons, New York (1987) p. 181-191.

174. Leveson, N., *System Safety Engineering: Back To The Future*. On line publication: http://sunnyday.mit.edu/book2.pdf(2002)

175. Lim, Y. Multiple Aspect Based Task Analysis (MABTA) for User Requirements Gathering in Highly-Contextualized Interactive Sys. Design. in *Tamodia*. 2004: ACM Press.

176. Lingard L, Espin S, Rubin B, Whyte S, Colmenares M, Baker GR, Doran D, Grober E, Orser B, Bohnen J, Reznick R., Getting teams to talk: development and pilot implementation of a checklist to promote interprofessional communication in the OR. *Qual Saf Health Care*, 2005. 14: p. 340-346.

177. Lingard, L., Espin, S, Rubin, B, Whyte, S, Colmenares, M, Baker, GR, Doran, D, Grober, E, Orser, B, Bohnen, J, Reznick, R., Getting teams to talk: development and pilot implementation of a checklist to promote interprofessional communication in the OR. *Qual Saf Health Care*, 2005. 14: p. 340-346.

178. Lingard, L., Espin, S., Whyte, S., Regehr, G., Baker, G. R., Reznick, R., Bohnen, J., Orser, B., Doran, D., Grober, E., Communication failures in the operating room: an observational classification of recurrent types and effects. *Qual Saf Health Care*, 2004. 13(5): p. 330-334.

179. Lingard, L., Reznick, R., Espin, S., Regehr, G., DeVito, I., Team Communications in the Operating Room: Talk Patterns, Sites of Tension, and Implications for Novices. *Academic Medicine:* , 2002. 77(3): p. 232-237.

180. Lutz, R. Analyzing Software Requirements Errors in Safety-Critical, Embedded Systems. in *IEEE International Symposium on Requirements Engineering*. 1993.

181. MacMillan, J., Entin, E. E., & Serfaty, D., *Communication overhead: the hidden cost of team cognition*, in Fiore, E.S.S.M. (ed.): *Team cognition*. American Psychological Association, Washington, DC (2004) p. 61-82.

182. Maier, M.W., Emery, D., Hilliard, R., ANSI/IEEE 1471 and systems engineering. *Sysems Engineering*, 2004. 7(3): p. 257-270.

183. Maier, M.W., Emery, D., Hilliard, R. *Recommended Practice for Architectural Description of Software-intensive Systems*. 2009 [cited July 29, 2010]; Available from: http://www.iso-architecture.org/ieee-1471.

184. Makary MA, Holzmueller CG, Thompson D, Rowen L, Heitmiller ES, Maley WR, Black JH, Stegner K, Freischlag JA, Ulatowski JA, Pronovost PJ, Operating room briefings: working on the same page. *Jt Comm J Qual Patient Saf*, 2006. 32(6): p. 351-355.

185. Makary MA, Sexton JB, Freischlag JA, Millman EA, Pryor D, Holzmueller C, et al., Patient safety in surgery. *Ann Surg*, 2006. 243: p. 628-635.

186. Malone, T.W., Crowston, K., The interdisciplinary study of coordination. *ACM Computing Surveys*, 1994. 26(1): p. 87-119.

187. Malterud, Kirsti, The art and science of clinical knowledge: evidence beyond measures and numbers. *The Lancet*, 2001. 358(9279): p. 397-400.

188. Marc-Thomas, Schmidt, The Evolution of Workflow Standards. *IEEE Concurrency*, 1999. 7(3): p. 44-52.

189. Marshall, S., Harrison, J., Flanagan, B, The teaching of a structured tool improves the clarity and content of interprofessional clinical communication. *Qual Saf Health Care*, 2008. 18: p. 137-140.

190. Mayhew, D.J., *The usability engineering lifecycle: a practitioner's handbook for user interface design*. Morgan Kaufmann Publishers Inc.(1999)

191. Mays, N., Pope, C., Qualitative research in health care: Assessing quality in qualitative research. *Brit Med J*, 2000. 320(7226): p. 50-52.

192. McRoy, S. W., Hirst, G., The Repair of Speech Act Misunderstandings by Abductive Inference. *Computational Linguistics*, 1995. 21(4): p. 433-478.

193. McTear, M., *Handling Miscommunication: Why Bother?* , in Dybkjær, L., Minker, W. (ed.): *Recent Trends in Discourse and Dialogue*. Springer Netherlands (2008) p. 101-122.

194. Medina-Mora, R., Winograd, T., Flores, R., Flores, F., *The action workflow approach to workflow management technology*, in *Proceedings of the 1992 ACM conference on Computer-supported cooperative work*. 1992, ACM: Toronto, Ontario, Canada.

195. Metz, C.E., Basic principles of ROC analysis. *Seminars in Nuclear Medicine*, 1978. 8: p. 283-298.

196. Mills, H. D., M. Dyer, and R. C, Linger, Cleanroom Software Engineering. *IEEE Software*, 1987. Sptember: p. 19-25.

197. Minoli, D., *Enterprise architecture A to Z: frameworks, business process modeling, SOA, and infrastructure technology*. CRC Press(2008)

198. Mishra A, Catchpole K, Dale T, McCulloch P., The influence of non-technical performance on technical outcome in laparoscopic cholecystectomy. *Surg Endosc.*, 2008. 22(1): p. 68-73.

199. Moorthy K, Munz Y, Adams S, Pandey Y, Darzi A., A human factors analysis of technical and team skills among surgical trainees during procedural simulations in a simulated operating theatre. *Ann Surg*, 2005. 242(5): p. 631-639.

200. Moss, J., Xiao, Y. A comparison of communication needs of charge nurses in two operating room suites. in *AMIA*. 2002.

201. Moss, J., Xiao, Y., Improving Operating Room Coordination: Communication Pattern Assessment. *J Nursing Adm*, 2004. 34(2): p. 93-100.

202. Moss, J., Xiao, Y., & Zubaidah, S, The operating room charge nurse: Coordinator and communicator. *Journal of American Medical Informatics Association*, 2002. 9(6S): p. 70-74.

203. Munkvold, G., Ellingsen, G., Koksvik, H., *Formalizing work: reallocating redundancy*, in *Proceedings of the 2006 20th anniversary conference on Computer supported cooperative work*. 2006, ACM: Banff, Alberta, Canada.

204. Muto, W.H., Israelski, E. Challenges in HCI Development for Medical Devices: A Human Factors Perspective. in *HCI Int.* 2005. Las Vegas Nevada.

205. Nagamachi, M. , Kansei engineering as a powerful consumer-oriented technology for product development. *Applied Ergonomics*, 2002. 33(3): p. 289-294.

206. Nemeth, C.P., Nunnally, M., Connor, M. F., Brandwijk, M., Kowalsky, J., Cook, R.I., Regularly irregular: how groups reconcile cross-cutting agendas and demand in healthcare. *Cogn Tech Work*, 2007. 9(3): p. 139-148.

207. Nemeth, Christopher, Healthcare groups at work: further lessons from research into large-scale coordination. *Cognition, Technology & Work*, 2007. 9(3): p. 127-130.

208. Nielsen, J., The Usability Engineering Life Cycle. *IEEE Computer*, 1992.

25(3): p. 12-22.

209. Nielsen, J., *Usability Engineering*. Morgan Kaufmann Publishers Inc.(1995)

210. Nielsen, J. *Medical Usability: How to Kill Patients Through Bad Design*. Jakob Nielsen's Alertbox 2005 [cited July 30, 2010]; Available from: http://www.useit.com/alertbox/20050411.html.

211. Nielsen, J., Rolf, M., *Heuristic evaluation of user interfaces*, in *Human factors in computing systems: Empowering people*. 1990, ACM: Seattle, Washington, United States.

212. North, R.A., Peterson, M.K. Improving Usability Engineering Through Post Market Usability Analysis. in *HCII*. 2005. Las Vegas.

213. Nyssen, A.S., Coordination in hospitals: organized or emergent process? *Cognition, Technology & Work*, 2007. 9(3): p. 149-154.

214. O'Cathain, A., Murphy, E., Nicholl, J, Why, and how, mixed methods research is undertaken in health services research in England: a mixed methods study. *BMC Health Services Research*, 2007. 7(1): p. 85.

215. O'Cathain, A., Thomas, K., *Combining qualitative and quantitative methods* in Mays, C.P.N. (ed.): *Qualitative research in health care*. Blackwell, Oxford, UK (2006) p. 102-111.

216. Ozarin, N. , *The Role of Software Failure Modes and Effects Analysis for Interfaces in Safety-and Mission-Critical Systems* in *IEEE Systems Conference*. 2008: Montreal.

217. Paek, T. Toward a taxonomy of communication errors. in *ISCA Workshop on Error Handling in Spoken Dialogue Systems*. 2003.

218. Paek, T., Horvitz, E., *Conversation as Action Under Uncertainty*, in *16th Conference on Uncertainty in Artificial Intelligence*. 2000, Morgan Kaufmann Publishers Inc.

219. Palmieri, P.A., DeLucia, p.R., Peterson, L.T., Ott, T.E., Green, A., *The anatomy and physiology of error in adverse health care events*, in Professor John Blair, D.M.F., Professor Grant Savage (ed.): *Patient Safety and Health Care Management (Advances in Health Care Management*. Emerald Group Publishing Limited (2008) p. 33-68.

220. Parker, S., Wall, T., *Job and Work Design*. Sage Publications, Thousand Oaks, CA (1998)

221. Parush, A., Kramer, C., Foster-Hunt, T., Momtahan, K., Hunter, A., Sohmer, B., Communication and Team Situation Awareness in the OR: Implications for Augmentative Information Display. *J Biomed Inf*, 2010. DOI:

10.1016/j.jbi.2010.04.002.

222. Pasmore, W.A., *Designing Effective Organizations: The Sociotechnical Systems Perspective*. Wiley, New York, NY (1988)

223. Paternò, F. Santoro C., Tahmassebi, S. Formal Models for Cooperative Tasks: Concepts and an Application for EnRoute Air Traffic Control. in *DSV-IS*. 1998. Abingdon Springer.

224. Paterno, F., Santoro, C., Fields, B. Analysing User Deviations in Interactive Safety-critical Applications. in *DSV-IS*. 1999. Braga Springer Verlag.

225. Patterson, E., Woods, D., Cook, R., & Render, M. Collaborative cross-checking to enhance resilience. in *HFES*. 2005.

226. Patterson, E.S., Cook, R.I., Woods, D.D., Render, M.L., Examining the complexity behind a medication error: Generic patterns in communication. *IEEE Trans Sys Man and Cybernetics*, 2004. Part A(34): p. 749-756.

227. Pepe, M.S., *The statistical evaluation of medical tests for classification and prediction*. New York: Oxford(2003)

228. Pinelle, D., Gutwin, C., Loose Coupling and Healthcare Organizations: Deployment Strategies for Groupware *J of Computer Supported Cooperative Work*, 2006. 15(5-6): p. 537-572.

229. Pinelle, D., Gutwin, C., Greenberg, S., Task Analysis for Groupware Usability Evaluation. *ACM Trans. Comp.-Hum. Interac.*, 2003. 10: p. 281–311.

230. Plasters, C.L., Seagull, J., Xiao, Y., *Coordination Challenges in Operating-Room Management: an in-depth field study*, in *AMIA*. 2003. p. 524-528.

231. Pocock, S., Harrison, M.D., Wright, P.C., Johnson, P.D. THEA: a technique for human error assessment early in design. in *IFIP TC 13 Int. Conf. Hum.-Comp. Interac.* 2001. Ohmsha IOS Press.

232. Pronovost, P.J., Nolan, T., Zeger, S., Miller, M., Rubin, H., How can clinicians measure safety and quality in acute care? *The Lancet*, 2004. 363(9414): p. 1061-1067.

233. Pronovost, Peter, Berenholtz, S., Dorman, T., Lipsett, P.A., Simmonds, T., Haraden, C., Improving communication in the ICU using daily goals. *Journal of critical care*, 2003. 18(2): p. 71-75.

234. Rasmussen, J., *Information Processing and Human-Machine Interaction: An Approach to Cognitive Engineering*. North Holland, New York (1986)

235. Rasmussen, J., Risk management in a dynamic society: a modelling problem. *Safety Science*, 1997. 27(2-3): p. 183-213.

236. Raymond, D., Process Improvement and the Corporate Balance Sheet. *IEEE Software*, 1993. 10(4): p. 28-35.

237. Reader, T. W., Flin, R., Mearns, K., Cuthbertson, B. H., Interdisciplinary communication in the intensive care unit. *British Journal of Anaesthesia*, 2007. 98(3): p. 347-352.

238. Reason, J., *Human Error*. Cambridge University Press, Cambridge, UK (1990)

239. Reason, J., Human Error: Models and management. *Brit Med J*, 2000. 320(7237): p. 768-770.

240. Reason, J. T., Carthey, J., de Leval, M. R., Diagnosing "vulnerable system syndrome": an essential prerequisite to effective risk management. *Qual Health Care*, 2001. 10(suppl 2): p. ii21-ii25.

241. Reason, J.T., *The human factor in medical accidents*, in Vincent, C. (ed.): *Medical Accidents*. Oxford Medical Publications, Oxford (1993) p.

242. Reddy, M., Pratt, W., Dourish, P., Shabot, M.M., Sociotechnical requirements analysis for clinical systems. *Methods of information in medicine*, 2003. 42(4): p. 437-444.

243. Ren, Y., Kiesler, S., Fussell, S., Scupelli, P., *Trajectories in Multiple Group Coordination: A Field Study of Hospital Operating Suites*, in *Proceedings of the 40th Annual Hawaii International Conference on System Sciences*. 2007, IEEE Computer Society.

244. Roseman, M., Greenberg, G., Building Real Time Groupware with GroupKit, A Groupware Toolkit. *ACM ToCHI*, 1996. 3(1): p. 66-106.

245. Rosenthal, M.B., Nonpayment for Performance? Medicare's New Reimbursement Rule. *New England Journal of Medicine*, 2007. 357(16): p. 1573-1575.

246. Roth, E. M., Christian,C. K., Gustafson, M., Sheridan, T. B., Dwyer, K., Gandhi, T. K., Zinner, M. J., Dierks, M. M., Using field observations as a tool for discovery: analysing cognitive and collaborative demands in the operating room. *Cogn Tech Work*, 2004. 6(3): p. 148-157.

247. Rothschild, J.M., Keohane, C.A., Cook, E.F., Orav, E.J., Burdick, E., Thompson, S., Hayes, J., Bates, D.W., A controlled trial of smart infusion pumps to improve medication safety in critically ill patients. *Crit Care Med*, 2005. 33(3): p. 533-540.

248. Roto, V., Mattila, K.V-V., Law, E., Vermeeren, A.P.O.S. User Experience Evaluation Methods in Product Development. in *INTERACT*. 2009.

249. Salas, E., Burke, C.S., Bowers, C. A., Wilson, K. A., Team Training in the Skies: Does Crew Resource Management (CRM) Training Work? *Human Factors*, 2001. 43(4): p. 641-674.

250. Sarter, N. B., Alexander, H. M., Error Types and Related Error Detection Mechanisms in the Aviation Domain: An Analysis of Aviation Safety Reporting System Incident Reports. *Int J of Aviation Psychology*, 2000. 10(2): p. 189 - 206.

251. Sawyer D, Aziz KJ, Backinger CL, Beers ET, Lowery A, Sykes, SM, et al., *Do it by design: an introduction to human factors in medical devices*. 1996, US Dept of Health and Human Services, FDA, Center for Devices and Radiological Health.

252. Scandurra I, Hägglund M, Koch S., Application of the multi-disciplinary thematic seminar method in two homecare cases - a comparative study. *Stud Health Technol Inform*, 2008. 136: p. 597-602.

253. Scandurra, I., Hagglund, M., Koch, S., From user needs to system specifications: Multi-disciplinary thematic seminars as a collaborative design method for development of health information systems. *J Biomed Informatics*, 2008. 41(4): p. 557-569.

254. Schultz, K., Carayon, P., Hundt, A.S., Springman, S.R., Care transitions in the outpatient surgery preoperative process: facilitators and obstacles to information flow and their consequences. *Cogn Tech Work*, 2007. 9(4): p. 219-231.

255. Seagull, F.J., Cheryl, P., Xiao, Y., Mackenzie, C.F. Collaborative Management of Complex Coordination Systems: Operating Room Schedule Coordination. in *Human Factors and Ergonomics Society Annual Meeting*. 2003.

256. Serfaty, D., Entin, E. E., & Johnston, J. H., *Making decisions under stress*, in Salas, A.C.-B.E. (ed.): *Team coordination training*. . American Psychological Association, Washington, DC (1998) p. 221-245.

257. Sexton, J. B., Makary, M.A., Tersigni, A.R., Pryor, D., Hendrich, A., Thomas, E.J., Holzmueller, C.G., Knight, A.P., Wu, Y., Pronovost, P.J., Teamwork in the Operating Room: Frontline Perspectives among Hospitals and Operating Room Personnel. *Anesthesiology*, 2006. 105(5): p. 877-884.

258. Sexton, J., Helmreich, R.,Neilands, T.,Rowan, K., Vella, K.,Boyden, J., Roberts, P.,Thomas, E., The Safety Attitudes Questionnaire: psychometric properties, benchmarking data, and emerging research. *BMC Health Services Research*, 2006. 6(1): p. 44.

259. Sexton, J.B., Helmreich, R.L., Analyzing cockpit communications: the links between language, performance, error, and workload. *Hum Perf Extrem*

Environ, 2000. 5(1): p. 63-8.

260. Skantze., G., *Error detection in spoken dialogue systems*. June 2002, Technical report, Dept. of Speech, Music and Hearing, Royal Institute of Technology, Stockholm.

261. Sorra, J., Nieva, V.F., *Hospital survey on patient safety culture*. 2004, Agency for Healthcare Research and Quality, Rockville, MD. Available: http://www.ahrq.gov/qual/patientsafetyculture/hospsurvindex.htm.

262. Spackman, K.A. Signal detection theory: Valuable tools for evaluating inductive learning. in *Sixth Int'l Workshop on Machine Learning*. 1989. San Mateo, CA: Morgan Kaufmann.

263. Spear, S., Bowen, H. K., Decoding the DNA of the Toyota production system. *Harvard Business Review*, 1999(September-October): p. 97-106.

264. Spear, S. J., Learning to lead at Toyota. *Harvard Business Review*, 2004(May): p. 78-86.

265. Stelfox, H. T., Palmisani, S., Scurlock, C., Orav, E. J., Bates, D. W., The "To Err is Human" report and the patient safety literature. *Qual Saf Health Care*, 2006. 15(3): p. 174-178.

266. Strauss, A. and Corbin, J., *Basics of qualitative research: Grounded theory procedures and techniques*. Sage Publications, Newbury Park, CA (1990)

267. Swets, J.A., Measuring the accuracy of diagnostic systems. *Science*, 1988. 240(4857): p. 1285-1293.

268. Swets, J.A., *Signal detection theory and ROC analysis in psychology and diagnostics: Collected papers*. Lawrence Erlbaum Associate(1995)

269. Taneva, D., Higgins, J., Easty, A., Plattner, B. Approaching the hotspot increases the impact: process breakdowns in a safety-critical system-of-systems. in *IEEE Systems*. 2009. Vancouver, Canada.

270. Taneva, S., Grote, G., Easty, A., Plattner, B., Decoding the perioperative process breakdowns: a theoretical model and implications for system design. *Int J Medical Informatics*, 2010. 79(1): p. 14-30.

271. Taneva, S., Law, E., *Interfacing Safety and Communication Breakdowns: Situated Medical Technology Design*, in *HCI Int*, Jacko, J.e., Editor. 2007, Springer Verlag. p. 525–534.

272. Taneva, S., Law, E., Higgins, J. Breaks in Continuity of Surgical Care: Considerations for eHealth Systems Design. in *Intl Conf eHealth Telemed Soc Med*. 2009. Cancun, Mexico: IEEE Computer.

273. Taneva S., Palanque P., Basnyat S., Winckler M., Law E., *Analysis of*

Communication Breakdowns for eHealth Systems Design, in *Nordic Conference on eHealth and Telemedicine*. 2006: Helsinki, Finland.

274. Taneva, S., Plattner, B., Byer, C., Higgins, J., Easty, A. Towards improving inter-team coordination in the surgical process: a breakdown detection method. in *ACM Int'l Health Informatics Symposium*. 2010. Arlington, VA.

275. Tang, C., Carpendale, S. A mobile voice communication system in medical setting: love it or hate it? in *CHI 2009*. 2009. Boston, MA, USA: ACM.

276. Taylor-Adams, S., Vincent, C., Stanhope, N., Applying human factors methods to the investigation and analysis of clinical adverse events. *Safety Science*, 1999. 31(2): p. 143-159.

277. Tellefsen, L., Failure mode effect analysis applied to hospital TB program. *American Journal of Infection Control*, 2005. 33(5): p. e162-e163.

278. Teng, S.H., Ho, S.Y., Failure mode and effects analysis: An integrated approach for product design and process control. *Int J Quality Reliability Management*, 1996. 13: p. 8-26.

279. Thomson, J., *Organizations in Action: Social Science Bases of Administrative Theory*. McGraw-Hill, Chicago (1967)

280. Van de Ven, A.H., Delbecq, A.L., Koenig, R. , Determinants of coordination modes of organizations. *American Sociological Review*, 1976. 41: p. 322-338

281. van der Aalst, W., van Hee, K., *Workflow Management: Models, Methods, and Systems*. MIT Press(2002)

282. van der Veer, G., van Welie, M. Task Based Groupware Design: Putting Theory into Practice. in *DIS2000*. 2000: ACM Press.

283. Vanderhaegen, F., Human-error-based design of barriers and analysis of their uses *Cogn Tech Work*, 2010. 12(2): p. 133-142.

284. Venkatesh, V., Bala, H., Technology Acceptance Model 3 and a Research Agenda on Interventions. *Decision Sciences*, 2008. 39(2): p. 273-315.

285. Vincent, C., *Patient safety*. Elsevier, London (2006)

286. Vincent, C., Neale, G., Woloshynowych, M., Adverse events in British hospitals: preliminary retrospective record review. *Brit Med J*, 2001. 322(7285): p. 517-519.

287. Vincent, C., Taylor-Adams, S., Stanhope, N., Framework for analysing risk and safety in clinical medicine. *Brit Med J*, 1998. 316(7138): p. 1154-1157.

288. Vortac, O. U., Edwards, M. B.; Manning, C. A., Sequences of Actions for

Individual and Teams of Air Traffic Controllers. *Human-Computer Interaction*, 1994. 9(3): p. 319-343.

289. Wainwright, M. *Shakeup after "lost" patient*. The Guardian 2003 [cited; Available from: http://www.guardian.co.uk/society/2003/mar/28/NHS.uknews1.

290. Wears, R.L., Perry, S.J., Wilson, S., Galliers, J., Fone, J., Emergency department status boards: user-evolved artefacts for inter- and intra-group coordination. *Cogn Tech Work*, 2007. 9(3): p. 163-170.

291. Wehner, T., Clases, C., Bachmann, R., Co-Operation at Work: A Process-Oriented Perspective on Joint Activity in Inter-Organizational Relations. *Ergonomics*, 2000. 43(7): p. 983-997.

292. Wetterneck, T. B., Using failure mode and effects analysis to plan implementation of smart iv pump technology. *Am J Health-System Pharmacy*, 2006. 63(16): p. 1528.

293. WHO. *Safe surgery saves lives*. [cited July 29, 2010]; Available from: http://www.who.int/patientsafety/safesurgery/en/.

294. Whyte, S., Lingard, L., Espin, S., Baker, G., Bohnen, J., Orser, B., Doran, D., Reznick, R., Regehr, G., Paradoxical effects of interprofessional briefings on OR team performance. *Cognition, Technology & Work*, 2008. 10(4): p. 287-294.

295. Wiegmann, D. A., Shappell, S.A., Human Error Perspectives in Aviation. *The International Journal of Aviation Psychology*, 2001. 11(4): p. 341 - 357.

296. Wieland, S., Brownstein, J., Berger, B., Mandl, K., Automated real time constant-specificity surveillance for disease outbreaks. *BMC Medical Informatics and Decision Making*, 2007. 7(1): p. 15.

297. Wiener, E.L., Kanki, B.G., Helmreich, R.L., *Cockpit resource management*. Academic Press, San Diego, CA (1993)

298. Willem, A., Buelens, M., Scarbrough, H., The role of inter-unit coordination mechanisms in knowledge sharing: a case study of a British MNC. *J Information Science*, 2006. 32(6): p. 539-561.

299. Wilson, R.M., Runciman, W.B., Gibberd R.W., Harrison, B.T., Newby, L., Hamilton, J.D., The Quality in Australian Health Care Study. *Med J Aust*, 1995. 163(9): p. 458-471.

300. Wilson, R.M., Runciman, W.B., Gibberd, R.W., Harrison, B.T., Newby, L., Hamilton, J.D., The quality in Australian health care study. *Med J Aust*, 1998. 169: p. 458-471.

301. Wilson, S., Galliers, J., Fone, J. Not all sharing is equal: the impact of a large display on small group collaborative work. in *CSCW*. 2006. Banff, Alberta, Canada: ACM.

302. Wong, H.J., Caesar, M., Bandali, S., Agnew, J., Abrams, H., Electronic inpatient whiteboards: Improving multidisciplinary communication and coordination of care *Intl J Medical Informatics*, 2009. 78(4): p. 239-247.

303. Woods, D., *Broad-based Systems Approaches*, in *National Summit on Medical Errors and Patient Safety Research*. 2000: Washington, DC. Available: http://www.quic.gov/summit/wwoods.htm.

304. Xiao, Y., *Understanding Coordination in a Dynamic Medical Environment: Methods and Results*, in McNeese, M., Salas, E., Endsley, M. (ed.): *New Trends in Collaborative Activities*. Hum. Fact. Erg. Society, California (2001) p.

305. Xiao, Y., Artifacts and collaborative work in healthcare: methodological, theoretical, and technological implications of the tangible. *J Biomed Inf*, 2005. 38(1): p. 26-33.

306. Xiao, Y., Hu, P., Moss, J., de Winter, J., Venekamp, D., Mackenzie, C., Seagull, F., Perkins, S., Opportunities and challenges in improving surgical work flow. *Cognition, Technology & Work*, 2008. 10(4): p. 313-321.

307. Xiao, Y., Hu, P., Seagull, F.J., Mackenzie, C.F., de Visser, J., Wieringa, P. Distributed planning and monitoring in a dynamic environment: trade-offs of information access and privacy. in *IEEE Int Conf Systems, Man and Cybernetics*. 2003.

308. Xiao, Y., Lasome, C., Moss, J., Mackenzie, C.F., Faraj, S., *Cognitive properties of a whiteboard: a case study in a trauma centre*, in *ECSCW*. 2001, Kluwer Academic Publishers: Bonn, Germany.

309. Xiao, Y., Mackenzie, C. F., Patey, R. Team Coordination and Breakdowns in a Real-Life Stressful Environment. in *Human Factors and Ergonomics Society*. 1998. Chicago, IL.

310. Xiao, Y., Mackenzie, C.F., Introduction to the special issue on Video-based research in high risk settings: methodology and experience. *Cogn Tech Work*, 2004. 6(3): p. 127-130.

311. Xiao, Y., Schenkel S., Faraj S., Mackenzie C.F., Moss J.A., What whiteboards in a trauma center operating suite can teach us about emergency department communication. *Annals of Emergency Medicine*, 2007. 50(4): p. 387-395.

312. Xiao, Y., Seagull, F.J., Emergent CSCW systems: The resolution and bandwidth of workplaces. *Int J Medical Informatics*, 2007. 76(S): p. 261-

266.

313. Xiao, Y., Seagull, F.J., Faraj, S., & Mackenzie, C.F., *Coordination Practices for Patient Safety: Knowledge, Cultural, and Supporting Artifact Requirements*, in *International Ergonomic Association*. 2003.

314. Young, T. P., McClean, S. I., A critical look at Lean Thinking in healthcare. *Qual Saf Health Care*, 2008. 17(5): p. 382-386.

315. Zala-Mezö, E., Wacker, J., Künzle, B., Brüesch, M., Grote, G., The influence of standardisation and task load on team coordination patterns during anaesthesia inductions. 2009. 18(2): p. 127-130.

316. Zapf, D., Maier, G. W., Rappensperger, G., Irmer, C., Error Detection, Task Characteristics, and Some Consequences for Software Design. *Applied Psychology*, 1994. 43(4): p. 499-520.

317. Zellermeyer, V., *Report of the Surgical Process Analysis and Improvement Expert Panel*. 2005, Legislative Assembly of Ontario. Available: www.ontla.on.ca/library/repository/mon/12000/256887.pdf.

318. Zhang, J., Johnson, T.R., Patel, V.L., Paige, D.L., & Kubose, T., Using usability heuristics to evaluate patient safety of medical devices. *J. Biomed Inf*, 2003. 36: p. 22-30.

319. Zhou, X., Ackerman, M.S., Zheng, K. I just don't know why it's gone: maintaining informal information use in inpatient care. in *CHI*. 2009. Boston, USA: ACM.

320. Zweig, M.H., Campbell, G., Receiver-operating characteristic (ROC) plots: a fundamental evaluation tool in clinical medicine. *Clinical Chemistry*, 1993. 39: p. 561-577.

www.ingramcontent.com/pod-product-compliance
Lightning Source LLC
Chambersburg PA
CBHW071409170526
45165CB00001B/219

* 9 7 8 1 4 6 1 1 1 1 9 1 7 *